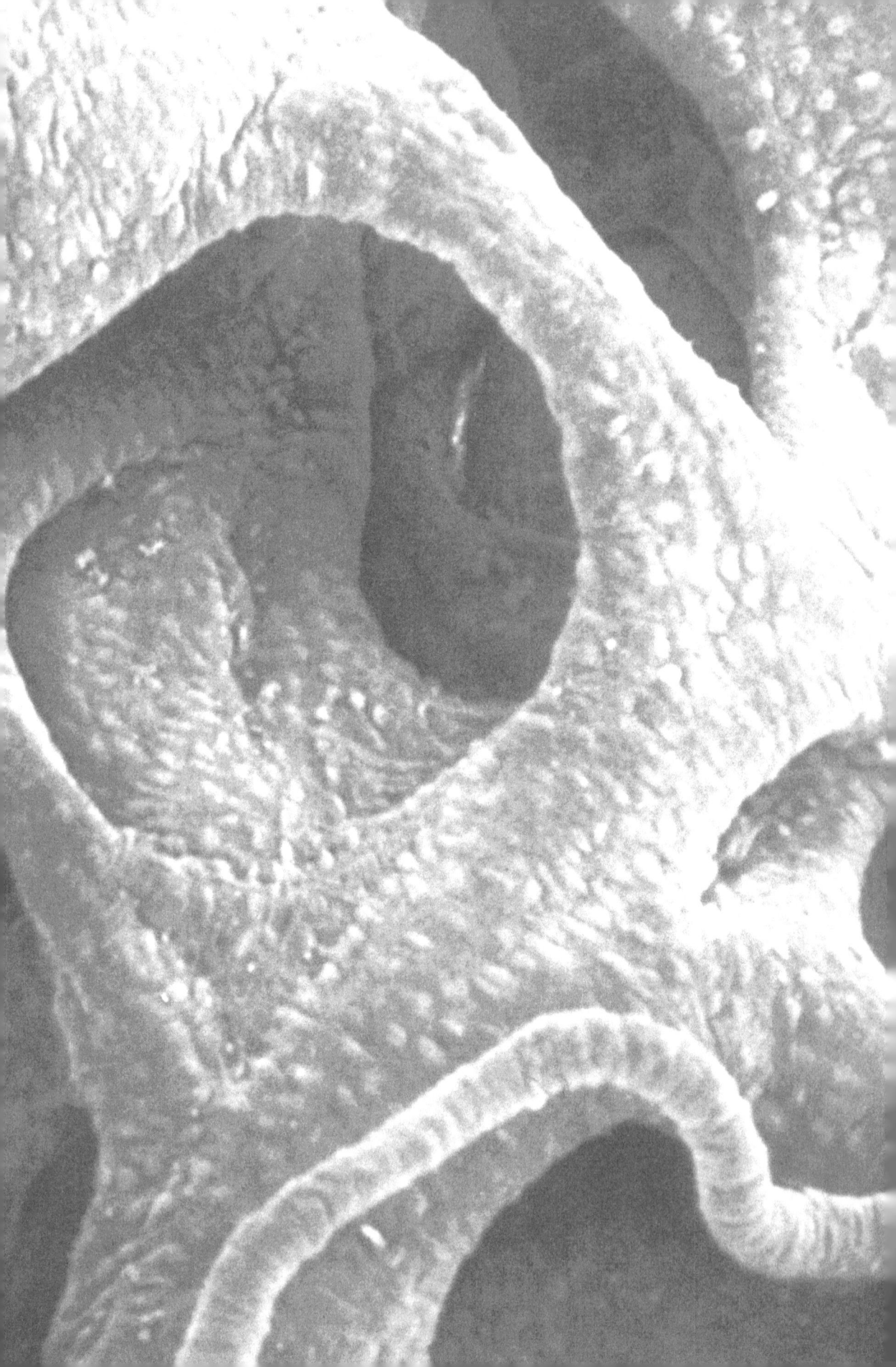

MEDICAL
INTELLIGENCE
UNIT

MONOCLONAL ANTIBODIES IN TRANSPLANTATION

MEDICAL
INTELLIGENCE
UNIT

MONOCLONAL ANTIBODIES IN TRANSPLANTATION

Lucienne Chatenoud, M.D., D.Sc.

INSERM U25, Hôpital Necker
Paris, France

Springer-Science+Business Media, B.V.

MEDICAL INTELLIGENCE UNIT

MONOCLONAL ANTIBODIES IN TRANSPLANTATION

Submitted: June 1995
Published: August 1995

© 1995 Springer Science+Business Media Dordrecht
Originally published by R. G. Landes company in 1995
Softcover reprint of the hardcover 1st edition 1995

ISBN 978-3-662-22197-6   ISBN 978-3-662-22195-2 (eBook)
DOI 10.1007/978-3-662-22195-2

Library of Congress Cataloging-in-Publication Data

Monoclonal antibodies in transplantation / [edited by] Lucienne Chatenoud.
    p.cm.
    Includes bibliographical references and index.
    ISBN 978-3-662-22197-6
    1. Transplantation immunology. 2. Monoclonal antibodies—therapeutic use. 3. Immuno-suppression. I. Chatenoud, Lucienne, 1956-.
        [DNLM: 1. Antibodies, Monoclonal—therapeutic use. 2. Transplantation Immunology.
        QW 575.5.A6 M746 1995]
    QR188.8.M66 1995
    617.9'5—dc20
    DNLM/DLC   95-24139
    for Library of Congress   CIP

Publisher's Note

R.G. Landes Company publishes five book series: *Medical Intelligence Unit, Molecular Biology Intelligence Unit, Neuroscience Intelligence Unit, Tissue Engineering Intelligence Unit* and *Biotechnology Intelligence Unit.* The authors of our books are acknowledged leaders in their fields and the topics are unique. Almost without exception, no other similar books exist on these topics.

Our goal is to publish books in important and rapidly changing areas of medicine for sophisticated researchers and clinicians. To achieve this goal, we have accelerated our publishing program to conform to the fast pace in which information grows in biomedical science. Most of our books are published within 90 to 120 days of receipt of the manuscript. We would like to thank our readers for their continuing interest and welcome any comments or suggestions they may have for future books.

Deborah Muir Molsberry
Publications Director
R.G. Landes Company

CONTENTS

EDITOR

Lucienne Chatenoud, M.D., D.Sc.
INSERM U25
Hôpital Necker
Paris, France
Chapter 6

CONTRIBUTORS

Daniel Abramowicz, M.D.
Department of Nephrology
Université Libre de Bruxelles
Hôpital Erasme
Brussels, Belgium
Chapter 4

Peter L. Amlot, M.D.
Department of Clinical
  Immunology
Royal Free Hospital School
  of Medicine
University of London
London, England
Chapter 3

Jean-François Bach, M.D.
INSERM U25
Hôpital Necker-Enfants Malades
Paris, France
Chapter 6

M. Cavazzana-Calvo, M.D.
INSERM U 132
Hôpital Necker-Enfants Malades
Paris, France
Chapter 5

A. Benedict Cosimi, M.D.
Massachusetts General Hospital
Harvard Medical School
Boston, Massachusetts, U.S.A.
Chapter 2

Alain Fischer, M.D.
INSERM U 132
Hôpital Necker-Enfants Malades
Paris, France
Chapter 5

Michel Goldman, M.D.
Department of Immunology
Université Libre de Bruxelles
Hôpital Erasme
Brussels, Belgium
Chapter 4

N. Jabado, M.D.
INSERM U 132
Hôpital Necker-Enfants Malades
Paris, France
Chapter 5

Anthony P. Monaco, M.D.
Division of Organ Transplantation
New England Deaconess Hospital
Harvard Medical School
Boston, Massachusetts, U.S.A.
Chapter 1

CONTRIBUTORS

John Powelson, M.D.
Massachusetts General Hospital
Harvard Medical School
Boston, Massachusetts, U.S.A.
Chapter 2

S. Sarnacki, M.D.
Laboratoire
  de Chirurgie Expérimentale
Hôspital Necker-Enfants Malades
Paris, France
Chapter 5

Mary Ann Simpson, M.D.
Division of Organ Transplantation
New England Deaconess Hospital
Harvard Medical School
Boston, Massachusetts, U.S.A.
Chapter 1

Michelle Webb, M.D.
INSERM U25
Hôpital Necker-Enfants Malades
Paris, France
Chapter 6

PREFACE

Polyclonal anti-lymphocyte antibodies were introduced in the early sixties and since then have proven to be essential tools to immunosuppress patients undergoing organ and bone marrow transplantation. Their use is, however, often limited by the lack of standardization and the difficulty of an adequate dosage adaptation. The advent of monoclonal antibodies directed at a vast array of functionally relevant T- and B-cell receptors has opened the way for a modern and more clinically appropriate use of anti-lymphocyte antibodies.

Experimental and clinical evidence presented in this book illustrates that antibodies expressing different specificities can be very effective in preventing or reversing established transplant rejection. Moreover, the data strongly suggest that the use of these new therapeutic agents may allow the induction of specific tolerance to transplant alloantigens.

It will perhaps not be long before tolerance becomes more than a sporadic and uncontrolled event after transplantation in man. This important goal, which seems likely to be achievable through the use of monoclonal antibodies, must guide and sustain the efforts and collaborations between basic scientists and clinicians in the field.

With great pleasure I would like to take this opportunity to thank all the contributors for their active collaboration and for sharing their experience in such a clear and up-to-date fashion.

Lucienne Chatenoud

CHAPTER 1

CLINICAL USES OF POLYCLONAL AND MONOCLONAL ANTILYMPHOID SERA

Mary Ann Simpson and Anthony P. Monaco

INTRODUCTION

The early attempts at clinical transplantation were effectively limited to kidney transplants and relied on non-specific immunosuppression based on steroids and cytotoxic agents. The resulting poor graft survival (approximately 50% at one year for recipients of cadaver allografts) sparked research efforts to develop improved immunosuppressive protocols which specifically targeted the lymphocytes responsible for graft loss and spared the recipient unwanted side effects. Two major areas of emphasis emerged: **biologic immunosuppressives** consisting of antibody preparations directed against lymphocyte surface proteins and **pharmacologic immunosuppressives** consisting of drugs whose major effects were on lymphocyte metabolism.

The introduction of cyclosporine-based immunosuppressive regimes into wide-spread clinical practice has resulted in markedly improved patient and graft survival. Recipients of renal allografts enjoy one-year graft survival rates approaching 90%. One-year survival rates for recipients of extra-renal organs vary between 70-90%.

Monoclonal Antibodies in Transplantation, edited by Lucienne Chatenoud. © 1995 R.G. Landes Company.

However, despite the improved early survival rates, the need for chronic immunosuppression remains and is associated with significant problems.

The most important of these problems is the failure of current immunosuppression to reduce the incidence of chronic rejection which accounts for the majority of late graft losses. Other complications associated with chronic immunosuppression include increased incidence of opportunistic infections and spontaneous neoplasms and drug-related side effects such as hepato- and/or nephrotoxicity and alterations in glucose or bone metabolism.

The focus of this chapter will be to compare the use and efficacy of monoclonal versus polyclonal antilymphocyte preparations in clinical transplantation. The major topics to be covered include production of the antibody preparation, use in the treatment of rejection, use in induction immunosuppression protocols either as adjunctive therapy or in cyclosporine-sparing regimens, side effects associated with administration of the preparations and, finally, use of antilymphocyte antibodies in tolerance induction.

POLYCLONAL ANTILYMPHOCYTE SERA

Antilymphocyte serum (ALS), antilymphocyte globulin (ALG) and antithymocyte globulin (ATG) are terms which are commonly used interchangeably although the products represent different degrees of immunoglobulin purity and result from the immunization of a heterologous species with different source lymphocytes. The most common source of lymphoid cells for the production of clinical ALG is human thymus; less frequently, thoracic duct or lymph node lymphocytes have been used as immunogens.[1] These sources of lymphocytes have the disadvantage of containing significant numbers of platelets and red blood cells which can lead to the development of immunologically irrelevant but potentially harmful antibody. Also, the precise composition of lymphocyte subsets within the thymus (or lymph nodes or thoracic duct lymph) may vary greatly between individuals so that these lymphocyte sources are incapable of presenting a defined, reproducible immunogen.

Attempts to overcome the lack of defined immunogen for the production of polyclonal ALS has centered on the use of cultured lymphoblasts.[2] This approach has the advantage of providing a consistent immunogen free of contaminating platelets and RBCs, but the disadvantage is that most stable cultured lymphoblast lines are B cells. The current availability of cloned T-cell lines may provide a superior immunogen for the production of polyclonal ALS, but the results of definitive clinical trials using this method are not yet available.

For experimental protocols, ALS has been produced in a wide variety of heterologous species and is frequently administered as whole serum. However, for clinical use, production of ALS is generally confined to horses, rabbits and goats, and whole serum is purified to the globulin fraction. The selected species is immunized with human lymphoid cells and, after an appropriate period of time, the sera is tested for antilymphocytic activity in vitro.[3-5] If acceptable activity is noted, serum is harvested from the animal and subjected to purification/safety procedures which generally include absorption to remove antibodies to platelets and RBCs, cultures to ensure freedom from viral and bacterial pathogens, and isolation of the IgG fraction from whole serum. The majority of ALS used clinically is produced by commercial enterprises (Upjohn Co., Fresenius, Merieux, etc.), but a few individual transplant centers continue to produce efficacious ALS products primarily for internal use.[6,7] Of note, it is estimated that only 2% of the antibodies present in polyclonal ALS/ALG are directed against lymphocytes.[8]

MONOCLONAL ANTIBODIES (MoAbs)

The intellectual impetus for the development of monoclonal antibodies came from the knowledge that a single B cell (and its expanded clone) would produce a single specific antibody. The means of translating this knowledge into a reagent with practical applications in clinical transplantation occurred when Kohler and Milstein successfully fused individual antibody-producing cells with myeloma cells, thus establishing permanent cell lines capable of secreting a single, defined antibody.[9] To produce the desired antibody, mice are immunized with an appropriate antigen such as a human T cell or a specific antigen complex such as CD3 in order to increase the number of cells responding to the desired antigen. Approximately one month later, splenocytes are harvested and fused to murine myeloma cells. The hybridomas are then grown in media which selects for their survival, the secreted antibody is tested for specificity and the clones producing the desired antibody are maintained and expanded. Expansion is generally accomplished by passage through the peritoneal cavities of mice or by sequential bulk tissue culture techniques.

Specific monoclonal antibody is purified from the ascitic fluid or culture supernatant and tested to ensure the absence of microbial pathogens. The nature of the immunization process and the specificity screening employed prior to clonal expansion preclude the development of antibodies specific to platelet or RBC determinants. However, new anti-lymphoid monoclonals considered for clinical use must be carefully tested to rule out cross reactivity with non-lymphoid cells (especially platelets, granulocytes and epithelial cells) as some functional surface proteins are shared by several cell types.[10] Between 90-95% of the protein in commercially produced MoAb preparations is specific antibody.

TREATMENT OF REJECTION USING POLYCLONAL ANTILYMPHOCYTE SERA

In the pre-cyclosporine era, standard treatment for renal transplant patients consisted of Imuran and prednisone as maintenance immunosuppression supplemented by high-dose steroids if acute rejection occurred. Rejection episodes were strongly associated with poor long term graft survival[11] and several transplant centers undertook controlled clinical trials to evaluate the efficacy of polyclonal ALS preparations in the treatment of acute rejection. The ALS preparations frequently were produced and used in a single center and the studies often involved relatively small numbers of patients, but they provided initial clinical data to document the effectiveness of ALS in reversing established cellular rejection.

Birkeland and colleagues[12] provided early data suggesting that ALG treatment was more successful than steroid therapy in reversing acute rejection, although in this series a long term survival advantage was not observed. Shields et al[13] conducted a prospective, randomized trial comparing ATG with high-dose steroids for rejection reversal in recipients of living related kidneys. They found that patients treated with ATG demonstrated a more rapid reversal of rejection, lower incidence of second rejections, better long term graft survival and function, and lower overall steroid requirements than the group treated with high-dose steroids. Similar results were obtained in another study involving recipients of haploidentical kidneys.[14]

Other investigators evaluated the efficacy of ALG in combination with high dose steroid for the treatment of acute rejection. Filo et al[15] compared ALG and high-dose steroids versus high dose steroid alone in patients experiencing a first rejection episode. Recipients of both cadaver and living related allografts were included and all received maintenance immunosuppression consisting of Imuran and prednisone. For cadaveric recipients, ALG plus steroid therapy resulted in a 91% reversal rate compared to 63% in the steroid only group. Better results were obtained in recipients of living related allografts, but again steroid only results were inferior to those in the steroid-ALG group (78% reversals versus 92%). Steroid-ALG combination therapy also resulted in significantly improved long term graft survival.

Clinical trials conducted by Howard et al[16] and Hardy et al[17] obtained similar results with superior reversal of rejection and long term graft survival observed in patients treated with both ALG and steroids compared to control groups receiving only steroids. A decreased rate of second and subsequent rejections was observed in patients treated with both agents. ALG was also noted to be a successful rescue treatment in a number of patients whose rejections were unresponsive to initial high dose steroid treatment.[17-19]

Cyclosporine-based maintenance immunosuppression became a standard feature of clinical transplantation in the early 1980s and has resulted in a lowering of the rate of renal allograft loss to acute rejection to < 20% in the first post-transplant year.[20] Nevertheless, reversible acute rejection episodes are still noted in approximately 50% of renal transplant patients. A somewhat higher rate is seen in recipients of extra-renal organs. Acute rejections that do occur in cyclosporine-treated patients appear to be more responsive to high dose steroid treatment than was seen with Imuran-prednisone-based treatment.[21] Among those CsA treated patients whose rejections are steroid resistant, approximately 85% will be successfully treated with ALG.[21-23]

TREATMENT OF REJECTION USING MONOCLONAL ANTILYMPHOCYTE SERUM

At the present time, the only monoclonal antibody routinely used in clinical transplantation is OKT3 (Orthoclone OKT3-Ortho Pharmaceutical Company). This MoAb binds the CD3 antigen present on all mature T cells and the CD3-OKT3 complex is then generally removed from the cell surface either through shedding or endocytosis[24] leaving affected cells incapable of normal immunologic responses. Initial administration of OKT3 also results in a rapid depletion of peripheral blood T cells. Clinical trial to evaluate OKT3 as an antirejection treatment quickly established it as a potent therapeutic agent equal to, and in some instances surpassing, the abilities of available ALG preparations to reverse rejection episodes.

Pilot studies were performed in renal allograft patients experiencing rejection while on Imuran and prednisone immunosuppression.[25-27] OKT3 was administered in doses ranging from 1-5 mg/day and resulted in reversal of initial rejection rates of up to 94%. A high rate of subsequent rejection was observed in these early studies (60-70%); this problem persisted until cyclosporine-based protocols became established. In cyclosporine-based regimens, between 60-80% of first rejections respond to high-dose steroids alone and approximately 85% of the remaining patients respond to a 10- to 14-day course of OKT3. Also, second or later rejections were seen in only 20% of OKT3-treated patients who were also receiving CsA.[28-30]

The primacy of OKT3 as first line treatment for rejection was established in a series of "rescue" trials in which patients whose rejections had not been reversed by addition of cyclosporine, high-dose steroids, and frequently ALG to prednisone and Imuran were treated with a 10-14 day course of OKT3.[30-32] High reversal rates (approaching 90%) were initially obtained in some trials, but high re-rejection rates were also observed and long term survival rates were relatively modest at 50%. In one series,[31] initial reversal was achieved in 74% of patients who failed ALG and steroids, in 67% who failed high-dose steroids alone, and in 71% who failed polyclonal ALS alone. One-year graft survival for this group was 64%.

Studies by Gaber et al[33] and D'Alessandro et al[34] demonstrated that regimens employing OKT3 early in the course of treatment for rejection were more effective at reversing rejection than regimens which reserved its use until other modalities had failed. They suggest a short (2-day) high dose steroid pulse followed by rapid introduction of OKT3 if steroid pulse is ineffective. This protocol appears to maximize the ability of OKT3 to reverse rejection while holding infectious and steroid complications to a minimum.

OKT3 has also been demonstrated to be an efficacious rescue agent for patients with extra-renal transplants who are suffering from steroid-resistant rejection.[35-37] Published reports suggest that these patients receive OKT3 treatment sooner relative to the time of clinical diagnosis of rejection and receive less steroid prior to its administration than kidney transplant patients. There is no evidence that these patient groups experience more severe rejections than renal transplant patients. It is more likely that this practice pattern is influenced by the lack of a dialysis-like alternative for these patients, and the probability that re-transplantation or possibly death are the only available alternatives should rejection treatment fail. Polyclonal antilymphocyte preparations are used infrequently in this group of patients and large multi-center clinical trials have not been reported.

ANTILYMPHOCYTE PREPARATIONS IN INDUCTION PROTOCOLS

The dramatic success enjoyed by both polyclonal and monoclonal antilymphocyte antibody preparations in reversing established rejection reactions has prompted a number of studies to determine whether these same drugs, given in the immediate post-transplant period, might act to prolong graft survival. These studies may be roughly divided into two categories. In the first group, the antibody is used as a cyclosporine sparing agent. The usual instance involves primary non-function of a renal allograft. The presence of OKT3 or ALG provides adequate immunosuppression, but allows the kidney an opportunity to recover from ischemic trauma without having to be exposed to the nephrotoxic effect of cyclosporine.

In the second group, the antibody preparation is added to obtain a perceived immunologic advantage. Potent anti-lymphoid preparations present at the time of transplantation would theoretically block T cell function and thereby prevent, delay or alter processing of donor antigen. These activities would prevent or delay rejection episodes and may facilitate the development of allograft tolerance.

Results of clinical trials conducted between 1983 and 1985 using ALG[38-40] or OKT3[41] for induction immunosuppression reported significant improvement in graft survival and reduction in number, severity and time to first rejection, as well as a decrease in the total number of rejections experienced. Similar results were obtained in the OKT3 Prophylactic Study conducted by Ortho Pharmaceutical Company which enrolled 224 recipients of primary cadaver allografts. Patients in the OKT3 arm (n = 117) received OKT3 (5 mg/day) on days 0-14, Imuran (2 mg/kg/d) and prednisone (0.5 mg/kg/day) beginning on day 0 with no cyclosporine until day 11. The control arm (n = 107) received triple therapy consisting of Imuran, high-dose prednisone with rapid taper, and cyclosporine beginning on the day of transplantation. Rejections in the OKT3 group were fewer in number, occurred later in time relative to date of transplantation and appeared to have a higher incidence of steroid-sensitive rejections when compared to the group receiving triple therapy. A trend toward prolonged graft survival was noted although statistical significance was not reached. The only surprising finding in this study was that the incidence of acute tubular necrosis requiring dialysis was the same in both treatment arms. This suggests that the delay in instituting cyclosporine therapy does not significantly impact upon the development of ATN and also argues against the premise that OKT3 administration is associated with increased incidence of ATN secondary to the release of cytokines.

Although several recent reports agree with the findings detailed above,[43-45] others have been unable to demonstrate a beneficial effect of prophylactic antibody administration.[46-49] Cecka et al[50] analyzed 3 year results from the UCLA-UNOS kidney transplant registry and found that prophylactic use of ALG or OKT3 was not affecting overall results in terms of graft survival or incidence of rejection. The first 1,000 transplants who received prophylactic OKT3 and the 3,000 first transplants who received prophylactic ALG were available for analysis. Graft survival rates at 1 and 2 years were only improved by 2% for recipients of either antibody preparation compared to recipients of triple therapy (Imuran, prednisone, CsA). Rejection in the first six months was reduced by 3% with ALG and by 5% with OKT3 with neither finding achieving significance in a multivariate analysis. This study did identify subgroups of patients that might potentially benefit from prophylactic antilymphocyte treatment. Patients undergoing second or subsequent transplants and those with delayed graft function did appear to have fewer rejections and better graft function at 1 and 2 years.

SIDE EFFECTS ASSOCIATED WITH ADMINISTRATION OF MONOCLONAL AND POLYCLONAL ANTILYMPHOCYTIC ANTIBODIES

Polyclonal and monoclonal antilymphocyte solutions are each associated with significant unwanted side effects (Tables 1.1 and 1.2). Some of these side effects are related to their physio-chemical composition and some to their mechanism of action. There is currently enough collective experience with these agents so that most of the clinically significant side effects may be anticipated and, in many instances, avoided.

Polyclonal antibodies such as ALG or ATG contain only about 2% specific antibody. Consequently, relatively large amounts of heterologous protein must be administered to the patient in order to ensure adequate amounts of specific anti-lymphoid antibody. The protein quantity is sufficient to elicit significant local inflammatory reactions if administered intramuscularly and may cause phlebitis if given intravenously into a peripheral vein with low flow. Therefore, most polyclonal antibodies in clinical use are administered intravenously, in a dilute saline solution, into a large vessel with good blood flow over a period of 4-6 hours.

The incidence and severity of adverse reactions associated with administration of ALG varies with the individual patient, the particular batch of antibody being infused and the species of animal used to produce the product. Of the species commonly used for the production of clinical ALG, most adverse reactions are noted with equine products and least with products of rabbit origin. The common side effects associated with ALG are noted in Table 1.1.

Table 1.1. Frequently reported side effects associated with administration of polyclonal antilymphocyte serum

Common (> 10%)	Occasional (5-10%)	Infrequent (< 5%)
Fever	Abnormal LFTs	Anaphylaxis
Thrombocytopenia	Serum Sickness	Hypertension
Rashes	Dyspnea	Hypotension
Chills	Diarrhea	Seizures
Leukopenia	Arthralgia	Deep Vein Thrombosis
Systemic Infections	Nausea	Perip. Thrombophlebitis
	Vomiting	Stomatitis
	Chest Pain	Pulmonary Edema
		Lymphoproliferative Disorders

Many patients (up to 80%) experience chills and fever during administration of the first dose and occasionally during subsequent doses. These symptoms are believed to be related to rapid lysis of lymphoid cells and consequent systemic release of pyrogenic cytokines (especially TNF, IFNγ and IL-6).[24] Dermatologic reactions are also noted frequently and presumably represent some form of delayed type hypersensitivity. None of these symptoms are usually severe enough to warrant discontinuation of treatment and most can be controlled or prevented by administration of antipyretics, antihistamines and, if warranted, intravenous corticosteroids prior to infusion of ALG.

Relative or absolute thrombocytopenia has been reported in up to 50% of the patients receiving ALG. The major cause of this is presumably antibody directed against determinants on the platelet membrane which are also on lymphocytes. Thrombocytopenia may occasionally be severe enough to necessitate termination of treatment with ALG.

Administration of OKT3 is less cumbersome than administration of ALG in that the usual daily dose does not exceed 5 mg and the preparation is supplied at a concentration of 1 mg/ml. An effective dose can be administered as a 5 ml i.v. bolus in 1-2 minutes, the preparation is not prone to aggregate formation, phlebitis and local inflammation are uncommon, as are dermatological reaction or cross-reactivity with platelets or other cell types.

Table 1.2. Frequently reported side effects associated with administration of monoclonal antilymphocyte serum

Common	Occasional	Infrequent
Fever	Rash	Asceptic Meningitis
Chills	Puritis	Lymphoproliferative Disorders
Rigor	Itching	
Nausea	Pulmonary Edema	
Vomiting	Myalgia	
Dyspnea		
Wheezes		
Diarrhea		
Systemic Infections		

Patients treated with OKT3 also experience symptoms related to cytokine release similar to that described for ALG following the first few treatments. It is usually more severe than that associated with ALG and may include fevers to 39°C, diarrhea and pulmonary distress. These symptoms occur frequently enough that patients are routinely medicated with antihistamines and antipyretic agents throughout their course of OKT3 and receive i.v corticosteroid in addition during their first treatment. As an added precaution, patients are routinely checked for signs of pulmonary edema and if necessary, dialyzed to ≈ 3% of their dry weight before initial administration of OKT3. Aseptic meningitis and vague neurologic complaints have also been noted but are not frequent complications.

Both OKT3 and ALG are prepared in heterologous species and can therefore elicit immune responses when injected into humans. Human anti-mouse antibodies develop approximately 2 weeks following cessation of treatment with OKT3[51] and if present in high titer can neutralize anti-CD3 activity and allow resumption of normal T-cell reactivity. Antibodies to ALG may also develop but are not noted with the regularity observed following administration of murine monoclonals.

Administration of both ALG and OKT3 is associated with an increased incidence of malignancy and viral infection when compared to patients who receive only double or triple therapy. Infectious agents of particular importance in this regard are the Herpes virus family which include Herpes simplex, cytomegalovirus and Epstein-Barr virus.[52] It is now well recognized that significant systemic infectious complications are most closely related to total amount of immunosuppression rather than to a particular type of immunosuppressive agent. As all antilymphocyte antibody preparations are potent immunosuppressives, most investigators now favor reducing the dose of other agents, especially cyclosporine, during administration of OKT3 or ALG. Concurrent administration of anti-viral agents such as ganciclovir or acyclovir during antibody therapy is increasingly reported.[53]

The malignancy most closely related to use of antilymphoid antibody therapy is the syndrome known as "post-transplant lymphoproliferative disorder." This results from reactivation of the Epstein Barr virus (EBV) and represents a wide spectrum of diseases. After the initial infection with EBV becomes asymptomatic, viral replication is inhibited by specific anti-viral T cells which eliminate B cells transformed by EBV. Drastic reduction of an individual's peripheral T cells as might occur with intense antilymphocyte antibody therapy creates a situation in which T cell control of EBV transformed B cells is sub-optimal. Multiple EBV infected B cells may undergo clonal expansion in this situation but, in most cases, antibody therapy is of short duration, and when T cells return to normal levels, elimination of virally infected B cells resumes. However, in situations where T-cell ablation is profound or prolonged, an increased incidence of malignant transformation occurs which renders expansion of the B-cell clone independent of EBV and impervious to T-cell control. This type of complication is seen most frequently in patients who have had multiple courses of antibody therapy and who have continued to receive full doses of cyclosporine and steroids during antibody administration.[54-57]

OTHER MONOCLONAL ANTIBODIES

Although OKT3 is the only MoAb currently in widespread clinical use, there are several other MoAbs that have had limited clinical use or are currently in clinical trials. There are several monoclonal pan-T-cell antibodies under development.[58-61] Unfortunately, none appear to be clearly superior to OKT3 in terms of efficacy, and most appear to induce the same spectrum of adverse effects and inhibitory anti-idiotypic antibodies following administration. An exception appears to be T10b9.1-A31, an IgM MoAb directed against the $\alpha\beta$ complex of the T-cell receptor.[61] Compared to OKT3, this MoAb demonstrated comparable ability to reverse rejection, elicited cytokine-related side effects less often and less severely, and was able to "rescue" a small number of patients who failed the initial treatment with OKT3. The implication with greatest clinical importance is the ability to effectively treat patients who failed OKT3, suggesting that future algorithms for clinical immunosuppression might benefit from the inclusion of more than one MoAb with the same general target but each directed at a unique epitope.

Monoclonal antibodies directed against the CD4 complex theoretically would disrupt normal antigen processing and consequently could be expected to have their greatest influence if present at the time of antigen presentation. A number of experimental models have confirmed this expectation and demonstrated that anti-CD4 MoAbs given at the time of transplantation resulted in significant graft prolongation and in some cases, specific tolerance to donor antigens.[62-64] Clinical trials have been conducted in patients with rheumatoid arthritis which suggest efficacy of anti-CD4.[65] Trials in transplant patients are currently underway but results are too preliminary to report.

An interesting molecular biology technique has allowed the construction of an anti-CD4 MoAb which does not elicit a strong antibody response in the individual being treated. In order to circumvent the inhibitory effects of anti-murine immunoglobulin antibodies which routinely develop following administration of MoAbs, a "humanized" version of OKT4A (anti-CD4) has been developed and tested[66] this molecule has a murine antigen combining site with specificity for CD4 grafted to human immunoglobulin molecules lacking antigen combining sites. The preparation does elicit anti-idiotypic antibodies but not anti-isotypic antibodies and has a significantly prolonged half-life compared to the native murine molecule.

Two other molecules have received considerable attention in the transplant community as potential targets for MoAb therapy. CD25 (IL-2 receptor, Tac) activity is required for T cell proliferation and for generation of cytotoxic T cell and antibody to this molecule results in significant, sometimes indefinite, survival of allografts in rodent models.[67] However, in higher mammals and in man, the ability of anti-CD25 antibodies to prolong allografts is not clear.[68-70] The second molecule in this category is CD54, an adhesion molecule also known as ICAM-1. This molecule plays a role in the access and egress of leukocytes into organs and has been implicated in reperfusion injury.[71-72] In a monkey renal allograft model, a monoclonal antibody to CD54 used a sole immunosuppressive resulted in significant graft prolongation.[73] A phase I clinical trial using anti-CD54 as adjunctive therapy in kidney transplant patients at high risk for delayed graft function reported improved graft function and survival compared to outcome of the contralateral kidney transplanted into patients who received standard triple therapy.[74] A multicenter trial using the antibody as adjunctive induction therapy is currently in progress, but the results are not yet available.

CONCLUSION

Advances in immunosuppression and organ procurement and preservation over the last 20 years have improved the survival rates of kidney transplants to 90% at one year and made transplantation a viable option for patients with end-stage hepatic, cardiac and pulmonary diseases. Cyclosporine-based maintenance immunosuppression protocols are efficacious and well-tolerated by most patients. A large percentage of acute rejection episodes are reversed by treatment with either polyclonal antilymphoid preparations such as ALG or monoclonal anti-T-cell products such as OKT3. Undesired side effects associated with administration of these biologic reagents have been well defined and reasonably controlled with appropriate medication at the time of administration so that very few patients are denied the benefit associated with the treatment.

Clinical and experimental research in transplantation has focused on targeting ever more specific components of the immune system with the ultimate aim of affecting the immune cell or cells responding to the allograft, while leaving the remainder of the system capable of normal responses. Clinical trials are currently being conducted with monoclonal antibodies against several molecules important in the normal functioning of the immune system, including some, such as OKT4A, which have been strongly associated with induction of tolerance on experimental models. Clearly, induction of tolerance to the allograft remains a highly desired outcome because, despite the significant improvement in 5-year allograft survival, most patients still face a future in which graft loss or poor graft function at 10 years is a probability. A review of tolerance induction protocols is beyond the scope of this chapter but it is possible to state succinctly that polyclonal and monoclonal antilymphocyte antibodies play a prominent role in many of the most successful strategies and, consequently, it is likely that antilymphocyte sera will continue to occupy increasingly important roles in future clinical protocols.

REFERENCES

1. Wechter WJ, Morell RM, Bergan J et al. Extended treatment with Antilymphocyte Globulin (ATGam) in renal allograft recipients. Transplantation 1975; 28:534-360.
2. Najarian JJ, Simmons RL, Condie R, et al. Seven year's experience with antilymphocyte globulin for renal transplantation. Ann Surg 1976; 184:352-359.
3. Gozzo JJ, Wood ML, Monaco AP. In vitro antilymphocyte serum cell-binding affinity as an indicator of in vivo immunosuppressive ability. Surg Forum 1972; 23:298-300.
4. Gozzo JJ, Wood ML, Monaco AP. Studies on heterologous antilymphocytes serum in mice. IX. In vitro assay by indirect leukoagglutination. Transplantation 1972; 14:358-362.
5. Gozzo JJ, Wood ML, Monaco AP. Indirect leukoagglutination: An in vitro assay for antilymphocyte serum. Surg Forum 1971; 22:277-280.
6. Thomas F, Cunningham P, Thomas J et al. Superior renal allograft survival and decreased rejection with early high dose and sequential multi-species antilymphocyte globulin therapy. Transplant Proc 1987; 19:1874-1876.
7. Hoitsma AJ, van Lier LH, Reekers P, Koene RA. Improved patient and graft survival after treatment of acute rejections of cadaveric renal allografts with rabbit antithymocyte globulin. Transplantation 1985; 39:274-279.
8. Monaco AP. Biological immunosuppression: Polyclonal antilymphocyte sera, monoclonal antibody, and donor-specific antigen. Organ Transplantation and Replacement 1988; 83-117, ed James Cerilli, JB Lippincott Co.
9. Kohler G, Milstein C. Derivation of specific antibody producing tissue culture and tumor lines by cell fusion. Eur J Immunol 1976; 6:511-519.
10. Latham WC, Cooney RM, Brown KJ et al. Preparation of purified antilymphocyte serum on an immuno-absorbent column. In Proceedings of a Symposium on Standardization of Antilymphocyte Serum 1970; 16:171-178.
11. Monaco AP, Codish SD. Survey of the current status of clinical uses of antilymphocyte serum. Surg Gyn Obstet 1976; 142:417-426.
12. Birkeland SA. The use of antilymphocyte globulin in renal allograft rejection: A controlled study. Postgrad Med J 1976; 152(Suppl 5):82-91.
13. Shields CF, Cosimi AB, Tolkoff-Rubin N et al. Use of antilymphocyte globulin for reversal of acute allograft rejection. Transplantation 1979; 28(6):461-466.
14. Nelson PW, Cosimi AB, Delmonico FL et al. Antithymocyte globulin as primary treatment of renal allograft rejection. Transplantation 1983; 36:587-589.

15. Filo RS, Smith EJ, Leapman SB. Therapy for acute cadaveric renal allograft rejection with adjunctive antithymocyte globulin. Transplantation 1980; 30(6):445-449.

16. Howard RJ, Condie RM, Sutherland DER et al. The use of antilymphoblast globulin in the treatment of renal allograft rejection. Transplantation 1977; 24(6):419-424.

17. Hardy MA, Nowygrod R, Elberg A et al. Use of ATG in treatment of steroid resistant rejection. Transplantation 1980; 39: 162-166.

18. Streem SB, Novick AC, Braun WE et al. Antilymphoblast globulin for treatment of acute renal allograft rejection. Transpl Proc 1983; 14:590-592.

19. Light JA, Alijan MR, Biggers JA et al. Antilymphocyte globulin (ALG) reverses "irreversible" allograft rejection. Transpl Proc 1981; 13:475-477.

20. Stiller CR, Keown PA. Cyclosporine therapy in perspective. Prog Transplant 1984; 1:11-29.

21. Matas AJ, Tellis VA, Quin T et al. ALG treatment of steroid resistant rejection in patients receiving cyclosporine. Transplantaion 1986; 41:579-583.

22. Richardson AJ, Higgins RM, Liddington M et al. Antithymocyte globulin for steroid resistant rejection in patients immunosuppressed with triple therapy. Transplant Int 1989; 2:27-26.

23. Benvenisty AI, Tannenbaum GA, Cohen D et al. Use of antithymocyte globulin and cyclosporine to treat steroid resistant episodes in renal transplant patients. Transpl Proc 1987; 19:1889-1891.

24. Chatenoud ML, Ferran C, Legendre C et al. In vivo cell activation following OKT3 administration. Systemic cytokine release and modulation by corticosteroid. Transplantation 1990; 49:697-671.

25. Cosimi AB, Burton RC, Colvin RB et al. Treatment of acute renal allograft rejection with OKT3 monoclonal antibody. Transplantation 1981; 32:535-540.

26. Goldstein G. An overview of Orthoclone OKT3. Transpl Proc 1968; 18:927-930.

27. Thistletwaite JR, Cosimin AB, Delmonico FL et al. Evolving use of OKT3 monoclonal antibody for treatment of renal allograft rejection. Transplantation 1984; 38:694-699.

28. Delmonico FL and Cosimi AB. Monoclonal antibody treatment of human allograft recipients. Surg Gynecol Obstet 1988; 166:89-96.

29. Thistletwaite JR, Gaber AO, Haag BW. OKT3 treatment of steroid resistant renal allograft rejection. Transplantation 1987; 43:176-180.

30. Norman DJ and Shield CF. Orthoclone OKT3: first line therapy or last option? Transpl Proc 1986; 18:949-952.

31. Widmer U, Frei D, Keusch G et al. OKT3 treatment of steroid and/or antithymocyte lobulin resistant renal allograft rejection occurring on triple baseline immunosuppression, including

cyclosporine A. Transpl Proc 1988; 20(Suppl 6):90-9-5.

32. Ponticell C, Rivolta E, Tarantino A et al. Treatment of severe rejection of kidney transplant with Orthoclone OKT3. Clin Transpl 1987; 1:99-106.

33. Gaber AO, Thistletwaite RJ, Ag BW et al. OKT3 as either primary or seconday treatment for renal allograft rejection. Transplantation 1987; 43:176-181.

34. D'Allesandro AM, Pirsch JD, Stratta RJ et al. OKT3 salvage therapy in a quadruple immunosuppressive protocol in cadaveric renal transplantation. Transplantation 1989; 47:297-301.

35. Cosimi AB, Cho SI, Delmonico Fl et al. A randomized clinical trial comparing OKT3 and steroids for treatment of hepatic allograft rejection. Transplantation 1987; 43:91-96.

36. Fung J, Iwatsuki S, Gordon R et al. Other organ transplant experiences with OKT3. Nephron 1989; 55:306-213.

37. Barr ML, Sanchez JA, Seche LA et al. Anti-CD3 monoclonal antibody induction therapy. Immunological equivalency with triple drug therapy in heart transplantation. Circulation 1990; 82(supple 5):IV291-4.

38. Novick AC, Braun WE, Steinmuller D et al. A controlled, randomized, double blind study of antilymphoblast globulin incadaveric renal transplantation. Transplantation 1983; 35:175-180.

39. Condie RM, Waskowsky KE, Hall BE et al. Efficacy of Minnesota antilymphocyte globulin in renal transplantation: a multicenter, placebo controlled, randomized double-blind study. Transpl Proc 1985; 17:1304-1306.

40. Sommer BJ, Ferguson RM. Three immediate post renal transplant adjunct protocols combined with maintenance cyclosporine. Transpl Proc 1985; 17:1235-1238.

41. Kreis H, Cjkoff N, Chatenoud L et al. Prolonged administration of a monoclonal anti-T3 cell antibody (Orthoclone OKT3) to kidney allograft recipients. Transpl Proc 1985; 17:2734-2737.

42. Monaco AP. Clinical aspects of monoclonal antibody therapy in kidney transplantation. Transplantation Science 1992; 2:9-13.

43. Ferguson RM et al. A multicenter experience with sequential ALG/ cyclosporine therapy in renal transplantation. Clin Transpl 1988; 2:285-290.

44. Goldman M, Abramowicz D, DePauw L et al. Beneficial effect of prophylactic OKT3 in cadaver kidney transplantation:a comparison with cyclosporine A in a single center prospective randomized trial. Transpl Proc 1991; 23:1046-1049.

45. Shield,CF. Effective induction immunosuppression for cadaver renal transplantation at the St. Francis Regional Medical Center. In: Terasaki PI ed, Clinical Transplant 1990. Los Angeles UCLA Tissue Typing Laboratory, 1990, 265.

46. Johnson CP, Simmons, RL, Sutherland DER et al. A randomized trial comparing cyclosporine with antilymphblast globulin-

azathioprine fro renal allograft recipients; results at 2.5-6 years. Transplantation 1988; 45:380-386.

47. Belitsky P, MacDonald AS, Cohen AD et al. Comparison of antlymphocyte globulin and continuous iv cyclosporine Aasinduction immunosuppression for cadaver kidney transplants; a prospective, randomized study. Transpl Proc 1991; 23:999-1002.

48. Matas AJ, Tellis VA, Quinn TA et al. Individualization of immediate post transplant immunosuppression: the value of anti-lymphocyte globulin in patients with delays graft function. Transplantation 1988; 45:406-412.

49. Michael HJ, Francos GC, Burke JF et al. Comparison of the effects of cyclosporine versus antilymphocyte globulin on delayed graft function in cadaveric renal transplant recipients. Transplantation 1989; 48:805-810.

50. Cecka JM, Cho YW, Terasaki PI. Analysis of the UNOS Scientific Renal Transplant Registry at three years - early events affecting transplant success. Transplantation 1992; 53:59-64.

51. Delmonicaom FL, Fullerm TC, Russell PS et al. Variation in patient response associated with different preparations of murine monoclonal antibody therapy. Transplantation 1989; 47:92-97.

52. Rubin RH, Cosimi AB, Hirsch MS et al. Effects of antithymocyte globulin on cytomegalovirus infection in renal transplant recipients. Transplantation 1981; 31:143-148.

53. Rubin RH, Tolkoff-Rubin N. The impact of infection on the outcome of transplantation. TransplantProc 1991; 23:2608-2609.

54. Penn I. Cancers complication organ transplantation. NEJM 1990; 232:1767-1791.

55. Malatack JF, Gartner JC, Urbach AH, Zitelli BJ. Orthotopic liver transplantation, Epstein Barr virus, cyclosporine, and lymphoproliferative disease: a growing concern. J Pediatr 1991; 118: 667-673.

56. Legendre CF. Effect of immunosuppression on the incidence of lymphoma formation. In: Roundtable Report:Immunosuppression and Lymphoproliferative Disorders. I. Penn, ed p. 11, Parsippany, NJ PRO/COM.

57. Swinnen LJ, Costanzo-Nordin MR, Fisher SG et al. Increased incidence of lymphoproliferative disorders after immunosuppression with the monoclonal antibody OKT3 in cardiac transplant recipients. NEJM 1990; 323:1723-1727.

58. Schlitt HJ, Kurrle R, Wonigeit K. T-cell activation by monoclonal antibodies directed to different epitopes on the human T cell receptor/CD3 complex: evidence for two different modes of activation. Eur J Immunol 1989; 19:1649-1653.

59. Frenken LA, Hoitsma AJ, Tax WJ et al. Prophylactic use of anti-CD3 monoclonal antibody WT32 in kidney transplantation. Transpl Proc 1991; 23:1072-1075.

60. Land W. Monoclonal antibodies in 1991: new potential options in

clinical immunosuppressive therapy. Clin Transpl 1991; 5:493-497.

61. Waid TH, Lucas BA, Thompson JS et al. Treatment of acute cellular rejection with T10B9.1A-31 or OKT3 in renal allograft recipients. Transplantation 1992; 53:80-85.

62. Cosimi AB, Delmonico FL, Wright JK et al. Prolonged survival of nonhuman primate renal allograft recipients treated only with anti-CD4 monoclonal antibody Surgery 1990; 108:406-409.

63. Sablinski T, Sayegh MH, Kut J et al. The importance of targeting the CD4+ T cell subset at the time of antigenic challenge for induction of prolonged vascularized allograft survival. Transplantaion 1992; 53:219-225.

64. Shizuru JA, Seydel KB, Flavin TF et al. Induction of donor specific unresponsiveness to cardiac allografts in rats by pretransplant anti-CD4 monoclonal antibody therapy. Transplantation 1990; 50:366-371.

65. Horneff G, Burmester GR, Emmrich F et al. Treatment of rheumatoid arthritis with an anti-CD4 monoclonal antibody. Arthritis Rheum 1991; 34:129-136.

66. Delmonico FL, Knowles R, Colvin R et al. Immunosupression of cynomolgus monkeys with humanized OKT4a monoclonal antibodies. Transpl Proc 1993; 25:784-786.

67. Kupiec-Weglinski J, Diamenstein T, Tilney N. Interleukin-2 receptor targeted therapy-rationale and application in organ transplantation. Transplantation 1988; 46:785-791.

68. Kirkman RL, Shapireo ME, Carpenter CB et al. A randomized prospective trial of anti-Tac monoclonal antibody in human renal transplantation. Transplantation 1991; 51:107-112.

69. Friend PJ, Waldmann H, Cobbold S et al. The anti IL-2 receptor monoclonal antibody YTH-906 in liver transplantation. Transpl Proc 1991; 23:1390-1393.

70. Soulillou JP, Cantarovich D, Le M et al. Randomized controlled trial of a monoclonal antibody against the interleukin-2 receptor (33B3.1) as compared with rabbit antithymocyte globulin for prophylaxis against rejection in renal allografts. NEJM 1991; 322:1175-1179.

71. Pober JS, Cotran R. The role of endothelial cells in inflammation. Transplantation 1990; 50:537-542.

72. Horgan MJ, Ge M, Gu J et al. Role of ICAM-1 in neutrophil mediated lung vascular injury after occlusion and reperfusion. Am J Physiol 1991; 261:H1578-82.

73. Cosimi AB, Conti D, Delmonico FL et al. In vivo effects of monoclonal antibosy to ICAM-1 (CD54) in nonhuman primates with renal allografts. J Immunol 1990; 144:4604-4609.

74. Haug CE, Colvin RB, Delmonico FL et al. A phase in trial of immunosuppression with anti-ICAM-1 (CD54) MoAb in renal allograft recipients. Transplantation 1993; 55:766-771.

CHAPTER 2

THE EXPERIMENTAL AND CLINICAL USE IN TRANSPLANTATION OF MONOCLONAL ANTIBODIES TO CD4 AND OTHER ADHESION MOLECULES

John Powelson and A. Benedict Cosimi

Monoclonal antibody (MoAb) technology has made possible the production of designer proteins specifically reactive with almost any conceivable biological molecule. The CD3 antigen was selected as one of the first targets for MoAb-based immunosuppression because it is present as part of the T-cell receptor (TCR) on all mature T cells. Disabling these cells, the pivotal actors in the alloresponse, was predicted to provide an effective approach to interrupting the rejection response in a more selective manner than that previously provided by polyclonal antilymphocyte preparations. The expected immunosuppressive effectiveness of anti-CD3 MoAb therapy has now been extensively confirmed in numerous clinical trials of OKT3.[1-6] Monoclonal antibodies reactive with other epitopes on the TCR have also been found to be capable of reversing allograft rejection.[7,8] However, suppressing all T cells

Monoclonal Antibodies in Transplantation, edited by Lucienne Chatenoud. © 1995 R.G. Landes Company.

indiscriminately increases the risk of infections and malignancies, while not necessarily being essential for effective immunosuppression. Suppressing selected T-cell subsets might provide comparably effective immunosuppression with less potential morbidity than these pan-T-cell reagents. Accordingly, MoAbs have been developed against targets such as the CD4 antigen, expressed on the T-cell subset involved in sensitization to the allograft (CD4[+] T cells); and the adhesion molecules, essential elements in the "second signal" required for T-cell activation. As predicted, these MoAbs have been shown to have potent immunosuppressive effects, including the capacity to produce donor-specific tolerance in animal models and are now undergoing clinical testing. Because of their remarkable properties, these MoAbs will likely play an important role in future clinical protocols and were therefore selected for review.

ANTI-CD4 MONOCLONAL ANTIBODIES

CD4[+] T CELLS

The CD4 molecule
   CD4 is a 55 Kd plasma membrane glycoprotein expressed on the approximately 60% of peripheral blood T cells that bind class II major histocompatibility complex (MHC) molecules.[9] CD4[+] T cells are equipped with an array of cell surface molecules mediating interactions with antigen-presenting cells (APC) (Fig. 2.1). In the classical immune response, a foreign antigen is first processed by host APCs, and then displayed inside the cleft of an MHC class II molecule. If a CD4[+] T cell has the appropriate specificity, the complex formed by antigen and self-MHC-II molecule is recognized and bound by the TCR. Closely linked to the TCR is the CD3 molecule, present on all mature T cells. When the TCR engages its target antigen, the CD3 complex transduces an intracellular signal that triggers T-cell activation. In the alloresponse, TCR recognition and binding also initiate activation; however, instead of foreign antigen in association with native MHC, the TCR now directly targets foreign MHC-II molecules.[10]
   The CD4 molecule projects outside the cell surface, where it can bind to non-polymorphic determinants of the MHC-II molecules on the surface of APCs (Fig. 2.2a).[11] This interaction increases the avidity between the TCR and MHC-II/antigen complex,

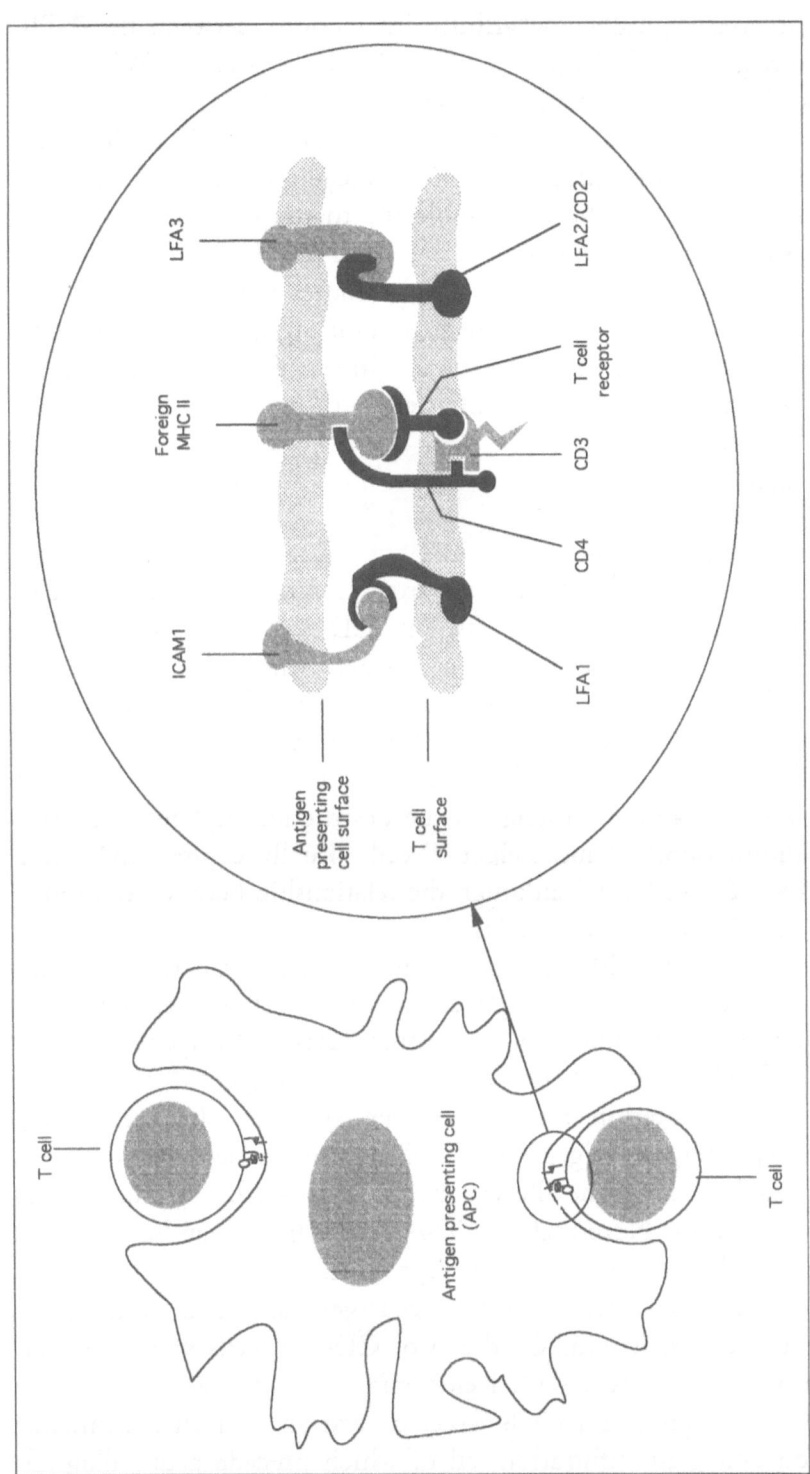

Fig. 2.1. T cell and antigen-presenting cell surface structures.

so that even typically low affinity interactions between the TCR and foreign MHC antigens are stabilized (Fig. 2.2b). When the extracellular CD4 domain interacts with the MHC molecule, its cytoplasmic tail is forced into close proximity with the TCR/CD3 complex. In this position, the CD4 molecule can amplify the signals transmitted by the CD3 molecule to the cytoplasm, thereby increasing T-cell responsiveness.[12,13] Thus the CD4 molecule has two functions: outside the cell, it promotes contact with APCs; inside the cell, it modifies transmembrane signals. Both functions tend to facilitate T-cell activation. MoAbs that bind to various epitopes on CD4 presumably interfere with one or both functions, and therefore interfere with CD4+ T-cell activation (Fig. 2.2d).

CD4+ T cells in rejection

CD4 and CD8 molecules are expressed on all mature T cells but in a mutually exclusive fashion. CD4+ T cells are generally classified as "helper" cells. When activated, they secrete cytokines which "help" activate other immune cells the effector cells. Effector cells, including cytotoxic CD8+ lymphocytes, the other major T-cell subset, and macrophages carry out the immune response that is responsible for foreign tissue destruction and foreign antigen elimination.[10] Thus, helper T cells usually express CD4 and cytotoxic T cells (CD8) although the relationship between cell function and CD4/CD8 expression is not absolute. An even stronger correlation exists with the class of major histocompatibility complex (MHC) antigens recognized by the T-cell subset. CD4+ T cells preferentially bind APC expressing MHC-II antigens, whereas CD8+ T cells bind cells expressing MHC-I antigens.[14,15]

In transplantation immunology, the correlation between T-cell phenotype, target antigen and T-cell function is less well-defined. Presumably because the alloresponse is so powerful, unusual T cell responses occur. Nevertheless, CD4+ T cells have been been shown to be mainly involved in the initial activation and amplification of the alloresponse, whereas CD8+ T cells generally mediate the ultimate tissue destruction. Of the two, CD4+ T cells would appear to provide the more essential elements of the alloresponse. CD4+ T cells are required for CD8+ T-cell activation, endothelial inflammation and graft infiltration, all of which precede acute allograft rejection.[16] Furthermore, CD4+ T cells alone can cause rejection,

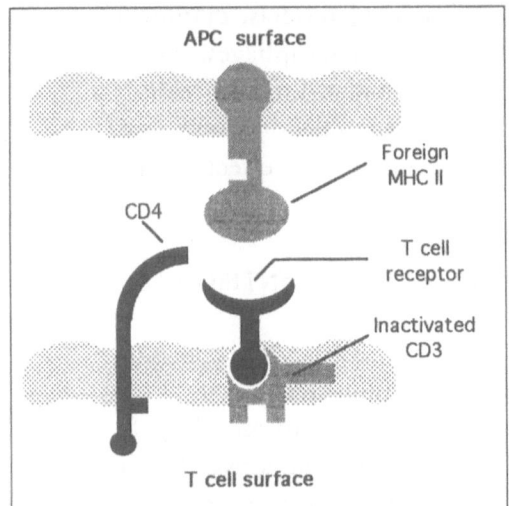

Fig.2.2a

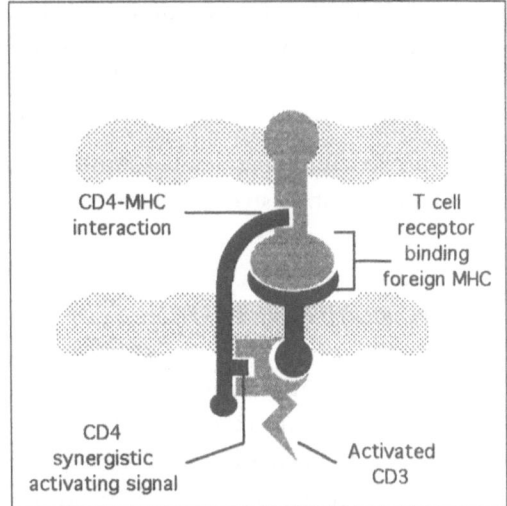

Fig.2.2b

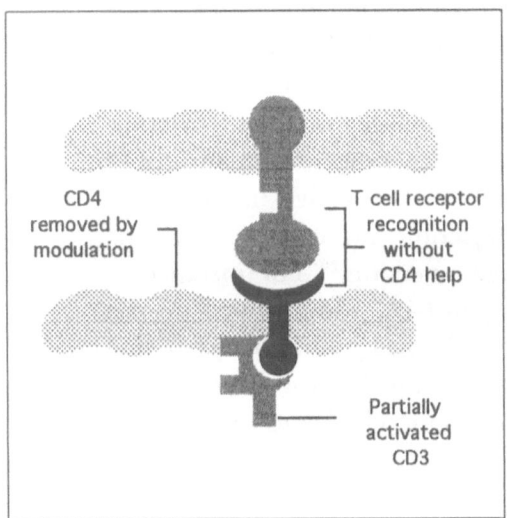

Fig.2.2c

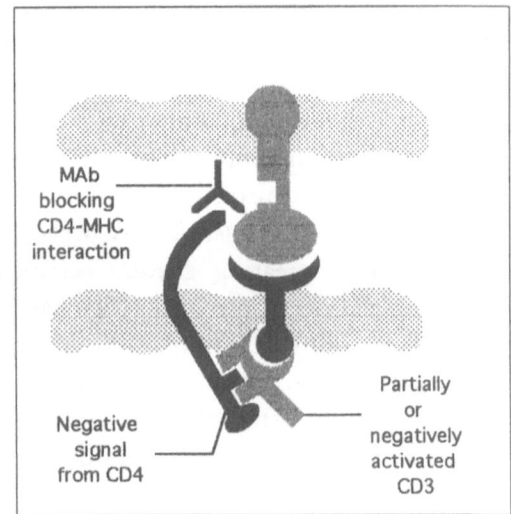

Fig.2.2d

Fig. 2.2. Modification of CD4⁺ T cell activation by anti-CD4 monoclonal antibodies. (a) Resting T cell. CD4⁺ encounters foreign antigen presenting cell (APC). (b) T cell Activation. While T cell receptor recognizes foreign MHC II antigen, CD4 binds it nonspecifically, resulting in a full activation signal. (c) CD4 modulation. Modulation by an anti-CD4 monoclonal antibody removes the contribution of CD4 to activation. (d) CD4 blockade. A blocking anti-CD4 monoclonal antibody can prevent normal CD4-MHC II interaction. As a result, activation is incomplete or even suppressed.

even in the absence of CD8[+] T cells.[17] In these models, cytokines secreted by CD4[+] T cells presumably activate macrophages, which then destroy the graft without the participation of CD8[+] T cells.[18] Because of the CD4[+] T cell's central role in the rejection response, interfering with its function is likely to provide an effective immunosuppressive strategy.

EXPERIMENTAL USE OF ANTI-CD4 MONOCLONAL ANTIBODIES IN TRANSPLANTATION

Anti-CD4 monoclonal antibodies: timing of administration

Given the role of CD4[+] T cells in sensitization to an allograft, anti-CD4 MoAbs would be predicted to be most effective during the early phases of the alloresponse, before effector mechanisms become self-sustaining. Observations in rodent transplantation models support this hypothesis. For example, naive rats treated for seven days prior to transplantation with BWH-4, an anti-CD4 MoAb, maintain a cardiac allograft for at least one month; in contrast, the same protocol employed from the day of transplantation is only marginally effective.[19] These results indicate that anti-CD4 MoAb administration is more likely to be effective in induction protocols administered to prevent rejection, rather than in rescue protocols treating already established rejection.[20] For instance, a single dose of the anti-CD4 MoAb OKT4A, administered on the day of transplantation, significantly prolonged kidney allograft survival in monkeys.[21] Accordingly, anti-CD4 MoAbs have usually been administered at the time of antigenic challenge in most experimental and clinical models.

Anti-CD4 monoclonal antibodies: mechanism of action

Depletion

Anti-CD4 MoAbs can be classified as depleting or non-depleting, depending upon their in vivo effects on CD4[+] T cells. Depleting MoAbs probably trigger complement through their Fc portion, resulting in lysis of the targeted T-cell population.[22] In most experimental models, CD4[+] T-cell depletion correlates well with the immunosuppressive effect of the MoAb. For instance, CD4[+] T-cell depletion from peripheral blood in rats significantly improved cardiac allograft survival, from 7.5 to 30 days.[19,23] Corresponding depletion of CD4$^+$ T cells occurred in graft infiltrates, which consisted only of unactivated macrophages and CD8$^+$ T cells. However, once CD4$^+$ T cells returned to the circulation, cytokine production and mononuclear cell activation were detected, and rejection ensued.

The clinical applicability of depleting anti-CD4 MoAbs may be limited because CD4$^+$ T-cell depletion has been unexpectedly long-lasting in several experimental models.[24-26] A single dose of an anti-CD4 MoAb in monkey kidney allograft recipients results in CD4$^+$ T-cell depletion to less than 10% of pretreatment levels. Although peripheral blood CD4$^+$ T cell levels return to about 30-40% of normal after 6-7 weeks, the cells remain depressed to about 60% of baseline for up to six months.[27] Similar results have been reported in patients, with depletion persisting for up to two years in one case.[28] Precursor lymphocyte depletion could theoretically explain this phenomenon, since immature T cells co-express CD4 and CD8.[29,30] The clinical consequences of this persistent depletion are unclear. Admittedly, CD4$^+$ T cells are also chronically depleted in human allograft recipients receiving conventional triple-drug immunosuppression, typically to 50-75% of pretransplant baseline.[31,32] Nevertheless, there is an understandable reluctance to add chronically depleting MoAbs to conventional regimens, and therefore it is questionable whether depleting anti-CD4 MoAbs can be successfully incorporated into clinical protocols.

Modulation

CD4$^+$ T-cell depletion, although highly immunosuppressive, is not required for anti-CD4 efficacy.[21,33,34] Some non-depleting anti-CD4 MoAbs exert their effect through CD4 modulation, a process whereby CD4 antigen expression transiently disappears from the cell surface. Modulation presumably removes any contribution of the CD4 molecule to T-cell activation, either as an adhesion molecule or as a signal transducing molecule (Fig. 2.2c). Modulation of the CD4 molecule can lead to significant delay of rejection in rats.[35] Similarly, modulation of the CD4 molecule in monkeys treated with OKT4A was associated with prolonged renal allograft survival.[21] In these animals, intragraft cells were found to be unresponsive to IL-2, suggesting that CD4 modulation prevents T-cell sensitization even in the absence of depletion.[36]

Blockade

Other immunosuppressive anti-CD4 MoAbs cause extended CD4 blockade, without depletion or modulation. This anti-CD4 immunosuppressive effect may result from interference with interactions between CD4 and MHC, or between CD4 and the TCR/ CD3 complex (Fig. 2.2d).[13] Like modulation, this interference might prevent the CD4 molecule from contributing to T-cell activation. Interestingly, CD4 molecule blockade appears even more immunosuppressive than modulation in some models. For instance, in a mouse model blockade was far more effective than modulation in improving cardiac allograft survival.[33] Since modulation presumably eliminates all CD4 function, the added effectiveness of blockade must depend on a different mechanism. It is therefore possible that CD4 bound by MoAb actually transduces a negative signal to the T cell, thereby suppressing its activation (Fig. 2.2d).[37]

TOLERANCE INDUCTION WITH ANTI-CD4 MONOCLONAL ANTIBODIES

The ultimate goal of transplantation is the induction of donor-specific non-responsiveness, which does not require continued administration of immunosuppressive agents. In this state, a genetically incompatible allograft is permanently accepted as self, while immunological responses to other foreign antigens are retained. The events occurring during the initial contact between host and allograft antigens appear to determine whether tolerance or rejection follows. Since CD4+ T cells are pivotal in the initial activation of the alloresponse, anti-CD4 MoAbs have been investigated for their potential to direct the alloresponse toward donor-specific tolerance rather than sensitization.

Striking results have been obtained in several rodent models. In rats, the pretransplant administration of the anti-CD4 MoAb OX-38, without any additional immunosuppression, achieved indefinite survival of cardiac allografts.[24] Animals with stable allografts showed specific unresponsiveness, since third party allografts were promptly rejected and responsiveness to immunogens encountered pretransplant was preserved. This specific unresponsiveness persisted even following removal of the allograft. Consequently, tolerance in this model is genuinely long-lasting, and not simply a functional consequence of continued low-grade antigenic challenge by the surviving allograft.

In another experimental model, whole blood was used as a source of donor antigen to induce tolerance to a subsequent allograft. Administration of donor-specific transfusions, together with an anti-CD4 MoAb, induced tolerance in mice to cardiac allografts transplanted 28 days later.[38] The advantage of this approach, compared with that of administering the MoAb alone on the day of transplantation, is that the nonspecific immunosuppressive effects of the MoAb have largely decayed by the time of transplantation. As a result, only donor-specific, rather than total, unresponsiveness persists at the time of surgery. Despite its appeal, this approach would not be applicable to cadaveric transplantation, where the timing of donor identification is not predetermined. To address this problem, further studies were performed to show: first, that a random blood transfusion given under cover of anti-CD4 MoAb immunosuppression leads to indefinite allograft survival; and second, that once established by random transfusion under anti-CD4 cover, unresponsiveness can be maintained for an extended period by random transfusions, without the need for further immunosuppression.[39] Even with these refinements, the clinical applicability of this model remains uncertain because of the possible risks of repeated blood transfusions.

Most of these tolerance models rely upon depleting MoAb. Because of the broadly immunosuppressive effect of CD4⁺ T-cell depletion, the exact mechanism of the tolerance induction has been difficult to elucidate. Non-depleting anti-CD4 MoAbs may also induce specific tolerance.[33,40] However, tolerance achieved with these agents has usually been to relatively weak antigens, or has been confined to specific strain combinations.[38] In these models, the CD4⁺ T cells are presumably rendered anergic when they bind donor antigen without a complete activation signal (Fig. 2.2d).[41] In addition, effector cells infiltrating the allograft may also be rendered anergic because donor antigen is encountered in the absence of the activating cytokines normally secreted by CD4⁺ T cells.[42] Interestingly, thymectomy prevents tolerance induction in some anti-CD4 MoAb models. It is possible that an intact thymus is necessary for the development of suppressor T cells responsible for tolerance induction.[4] Alternatively, new thymic migrants may be rendered anergic upon encountering antigen in the periphery if help from CD4⁺ T cells is unavailable.[44]

PRECLINICAL AND CLINICAL USE OF ANTI-CD4 MONOCLONAL
ANTIBODIES

Nonhuman primate models of anti-CD4 therapy

The striking results of anti-CD4 immunotherapy in rodent
models led to background preclinical studies in nonhuman primates.[21] To simulate the clinical situation, cynomolgus recipients
of renal allografts were paired with donor monkeys on the basis of
MHC class I and II mismatching. Recipients were treated with
OKT4A, a murine IgG2a anti-human CD4 MoAb crossreactive
with cynomolgus CD4 antigen. The MoAb was administered as
the sole immunosuppressant, either as a single high-dose
(10 mg/kg) pretransplant bolus, or as repeated low-dose (0.3 mg/kg)
treatments, begun pretransplant and continued daily for a total of
12 doses. With both regimens, CD4 coating and modulation were
observed, and significant prolongation of kidney allograft survival
resulted (Table 2.1).

Despite the dramatic efficacy of murine OKT4A immunotherapy in these monkeys, two significant differences from the rodent model observations were apparent. First, allograft rejection,
though delayed, eventually occurred in all OKT4A-treated recipi-

*Table 2.1. Immunosuppressive efficacy of murine IgG2a OKT4A, and of
CDR-grafted IgG1 and IgG4 OKT4A in cynomolgus renal allograft
recipients[27]*

Group	n	Onset of Rejection (days)	Allograft Survival (days)
Control	4	5.5 ± 0.7	9.0 ± 0.7
Murine OKT4A (IgG2a)			
0.3 mg/kg/day x12	10	16.9 ± 3.1*	25.4 ± 4.3*
10 mg/kg x1	5	30.8 ± 7.1*	39.0 ± 6.4*
CDR-grafted OKT4A (IgG1)			
1 mg/kg/day x12	2	25.0 ± 3.0*	39.0 ± 5.0*
10 mg/kg x1	5	35.4 ± 5.5*	45.2 ± 6.0*
CDR-grafted OKT4A (IgG4)			
1 mg/kg/day x12	2	13.0 ± 6.0	15.5 ± 6.5
10 mg/kg x1	3	24.7 ± 4.9*	35.3 ± 7.2*

* p < 0.05 versus control.

ents; and second, all monkey recipients of OKT4A developed anti-mouse antibodies. Thus, the clinical application of induction protocols including OKT4A could limit the subsequent use of other murine MoAbs. To address these problems, humanized versions of OKT4A were developed. In the modified OKT4A, only the original murine complementarity determining regions (CDR) were preserved (Fig. 2.3). Since these regions bind the target antigen on CD4, the original specificity of OKT4A was preserved. The remainder of the original murine MoAb molecule was completely humanized. To accomplish this, its CDRs were grafted onto a human variable region framework, and the resultant structure was then combined with either a human IgG1 or IgG4 constant region.[45-47] These isotypes were selected because of documented differences in their effector function: human IgG1 antibodies activate complement, with resultant target lysis, whereas IgG4 antibodies do not.[22] The objectives for humanizing OKT4A were to reduce its immunogenicity and, hopefully, provide a molecule which could more efficiently recruit the immunologic mechanisms required for CD4+ T-cell inactivation in both monkey and human allograft recipients.

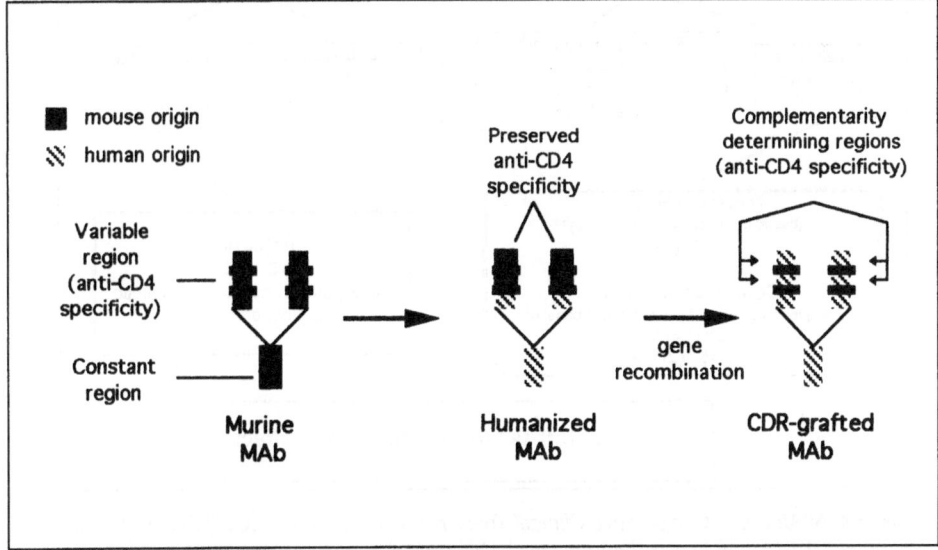

Fig. 2.3. CDR-grafted OKT4A. The murine OKT4A is progressively humanized, so that only the original complementarity determining regions (CDR) remain. These CDRs specifically bind the CD4 target.

Both OKTcdr4A MoAbs have been tested in cynomolgus monkeys, in a model analogous to that used to test the murine version.[27] Whereas CD4 antigen coating and modulation had been observed with the murine IgG2a OKT4A, only MoAb coating of CD4[+] T cells occurred with the IgG4 OKTcdr4A. Consistent and prolonged CD4[+] T-cell depletion was observed following IgG1 OKTcdr4A administration. The OKTcdr4A MoAbs retained the immunosuppressive potency of the murine MoAb (Table 2.1); however, their immunogenicity was reduced, and recipient serum levels were maintained for a longer period than following treat-

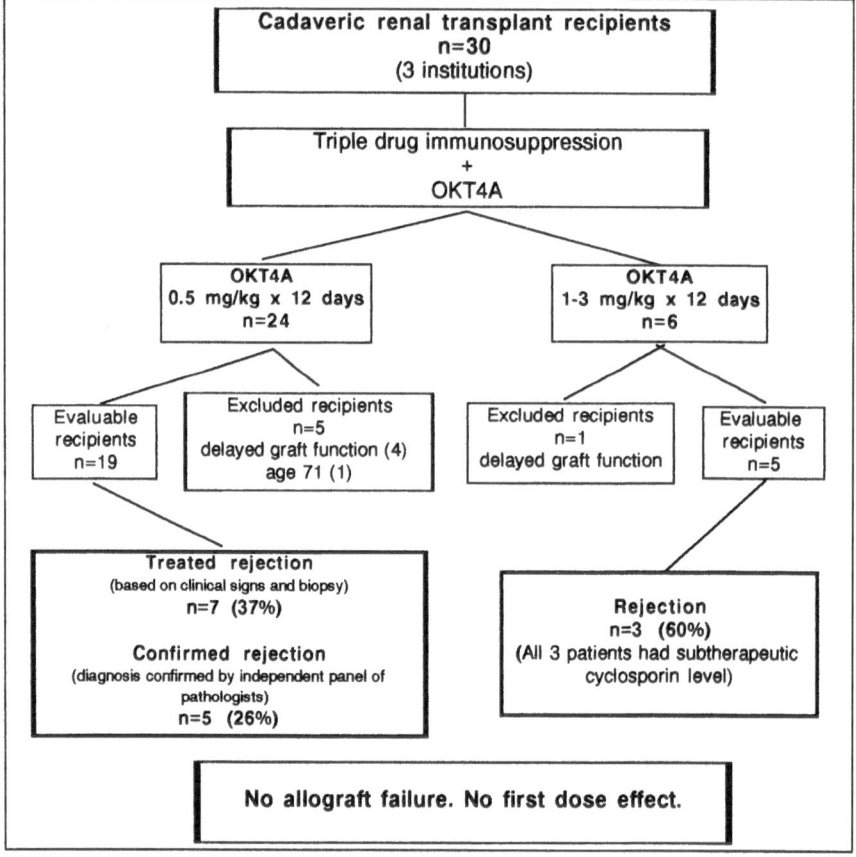

Fig. 2.4. *NIAID/NIH Cooperative Clinical Trials in Transplantation (CCTT) Phase I trial of murine OKT4A. Safety was demonstrated. Differences in biopsy interpretation between center pathologists and CCTT panel underscore the difficulty in using rejection treatment as a primary outcome, in the absence of investigator masking.*

ment with murine preparation.[48] The anti-MoAb antibodies detected following OKTcdr4A administration crossreacted only to murine IgG2a OKT4A, but not to other IgG2a and IgG1 MoAbs. This anti-MoAb response, presumably restricted to the original CDR, should not preclude sequential therapy with MoAbs targeting different epitopes, e.g. OKT3. Thus, a single pretransplant bolus of a OKTcdr4A MoAb could provide simple and effective induction therapy, without limiting the opportunity for possibly needed subsequent anti-rejection therapy.

CLINICAL TRIALS OF ANTI-CD4 THERAPY

OKT4A

A pilot study of murine OKT4A was conducted in cadaveric renal allograft recipients by the NIAID/NIH sponsored Cooperative Trials in Transplantation (CCTT) (Delmonico, in press). In addition to cyclosporin, azathioprine and prednisone, OKT4A was administered for 12 consecutive days, beginning on the day of transplant. Results are detailed in Figure 2.4. The absence of allograft failure or side-effects, and the observation of a three-month rejection rate of 37% (all treated), or 26% (confirmed) in patients treated with the 0.5 mg/kg dose of OKTA support the continued investigation of the anti-CD4 approach to immunotherapy. The next phase will be to test OKTcdr4A MoAbs in human patients. Because of the theoretical disadvantage of prolonged depletion, the nondepleting IgG4 CDR-grafted MoAb has been selected for the initial pilot study, which is in progress.

cM-T412

Another humanized anti-CD4 MoAb, cM-T412, has been tested in cardiac allograft recipients.[49] The MoAb was administered intraoperatively and on postoperative days 1-7, 9, 11, 13, 17 and 21. Compared to a control group treated with antithymocyte globulin (ATG), patients who received cM-T412 had fewer and significantly delayed rejection episodes and better overall survival (Table 2.2). Interestingly, fewer infections occurred in the experimental group, despite long-lasting T-cell depletion. These preliminary observations have encouraged more extensive studies which are currently underway.

Other anti-CD4 monoclonal antibodies

The anti-CD4 MoAb, Max.16H5, was initially found to be effective in patients with rheumatoid arthritis.[50] In renal allograft recipients suffering late-onset rejection, 16H5 was shown to dramatically deplete CD4$^+$ T cells, improve allograft function and eliminate the histopathologic features of rejection in the majority of treated patients. In addition, neither anti-isotypic nor anti-idiotypic antibodies to Max.16H5 were detected in any of the recipients.[51] Interestingly, reversal of established rejection would not have been predicted from the presumed mechanism of action of anti-CD4 MoAbs (see above: *Timing of administration*). Despite these compelling results, further trials with this MoAb have been limited. Trials in renal allograft recipients of other anti-CD4 MoAbs, e.g., BL4 and MT151, have not been as encouraging.[52,53] Even with transient CD4 depletion and the concomitant administration of conventional immunosuppression, the incidence of early rejection was unexpectedly high in these recipients (over 50%), discouraging further studies. Nevertheless, these multiple clinical trials emphasize the intense interest in immunosuppression using anti-CD4 MoAbs. The results observed in rodent and some non-human primate models suggest that these agents will almost surely play a prominent role in future clinical immunosuppressive protocols.

MONOCLONAL ANTIBODIES TO ADHESION MOLECULES

Acute rejection of histoincompatible tissues resembles a well-orchestrated assault by successive waves of host cells. Within hours of engraftment, perivascular infiltrates of host lymphocytes appear. A few days later, numerous, predominantly T, host cells scatter throughout the graft. Increasing numbers of phagocytic mononuclear cells then gradually enter the graft, resulting in progressive tissue disruption and subsequent graft necrosis.[54] This infiltration by sequential cell populations is characteristic of acute rejection. Interestingly, an inflammatory infiltrate is also the histological hallmark of ischemic reperfusion injury.[55] Thus, cellular infiltration occurs in the two most important causes of allograft injury. Consequently, an important goal of transplantation immunology is to define both the mechanisms that govern these infiltrates and possible approaches to their modification.

As a barrier between blood and parenchyma, the endothelium is well-positioned to regulate cellular migration from the circulation into tissues.[56] The endothelial cell apparently recruits infiltrating cells by expressing adhesion molecules on its surface. In addition, these adhesion molecules play an essential role in providing the accessory signals required for optimal activation of antigen-stimulated cells. Accordingly, disabling these adhesion molecules with MoAbs should inhibit proliferative and cytotoxic T-cell function, and limit any inflammatory phenomena associated with cellular infiltration. For transplantation, such MoAbs could provide the highly desirable benefit of simultaneously interrupting both the alloresponse and the effects of ischemic injury. Some MoAbs have indeed shown this dual promise and are now the subject of intense investigations.

Adhesion Molecules

Based on their structure, adhesion molecules in the immune system are grouped into three classes: selectins, integrins and immunoglobulins.

Selectins are small glycoproteins with a lectin domain and an epidermal growth factor-like motif (Table 2.3). Their structure is well-adapted for binding surface carbohydrate ligands.[57,58] Activated endothelial cells express P- and E-selectins, which mediate contact with neutrophils and lymphocytes respectively.[59] L-selectin, which is mainly expressed on neutrophils, monocytes and T cells, interacts

---

Table 2.2. Anti-CD4 immunosuppression in heart transplant patients

	cM-T412 + Triple Immunosuppression	ATG + Triple Immunosuppression
Acute rejection episodes (per 100 patient days)	.26	.41
Time to 1st rejection (days)	43.7	25.3
Episodes of infections (per 100 patient days)	.49	.91
1-year survival (%)	91	73

Results with cM-T412, a chimerized anti-CD4 monoclonal antibody, used as an adjunct to standard triple drug immunosuppression in the early postoperative period in heart transplant patients. Treated patients had fewer and significantly delayed rejection episodes, better overall survival, and fewer infections.[49]

with the endothelial cell surface.[60] In general, selectins mediate the initial weak binding between endothelial cells and leukocytes, setting the stage for stronger binding by other adhesion molecules.[61]

Integrins are much larger molecules than selectins, composed of two noncovalently linked a and b polypeptide chains, each of which has a CD designation (Table 2.4). Because they span the cellular membrane, integrins are well-adapted to coordinate extracellular contacts with intracellular events.[61] Thus, while the outer domains bind target proteins, the cytoplasmic tails interact with the cell's cytoskeleton to induce changes in shape and motility. As a result, integrins play an important role in regulating the sequential adhesion and de-adhesion required for cellular migration into tissues. The integrin LFA-1 (CD11a-CD18), which is present on lymphocytes, granulocytes and monocytes series,[62] is of particular interest as a possible target for MoAb therapy.

Table 2.3. Selectins [60, 63, 65]

Selectin	Distribution	Ligand	Comment
E-selectin (CD62E)	Activated endothelium	Sialylated glycoprotein on granulocytes and lymphocytes	Mediates binding of resting CD4+ memory T cell subset. Probably involved in neutrophil rolling.
P-selectin (CD62P)	Platelet, megakaryocytes, endothelium	Sialylated glycoprotein on myeloid cells and lymphocytes	
L-selectin (CD62L)	All leukocytes	Sialylated glycoprotein on high endothelial venule and inflammed endothelium	Peripheral lymph node homing receptor, mediates neutrophil rolling

In the immunoglobulin supergene family, which includes the TCR, MHC I and II, CD4, CD8 and CD3, evolution has preserved one or more Ig domains (Table 2.5). The intercellular adhesion molecules (ICAM-1 and ICAM-2) also belong to this family, and are detected on a wide variety of cells, including endothelial cells and leukocytes. Resting cells only express small amounts of these ligands on their surface, but inflammation or early antigen recognition leads to a dramatic upregulation.[61] In general, adhesion molecules in this family either bind integrins or other members of the immunoglobulin supergene family. The ICAM molecules, being ligands for LFA-1, are also attractive targets for immunosuppressive therapy.

CELL MIGRATION INTO TISSUES

This somewhat bewildering array of adhesion molecules is apparently required to coordinate the normal movement of multiple cell populations moving through the circulation, tissues and lymphatics. These adhesion molecules also regulate cellular migration into an inflammatory focus. Much like coagulation, the inflammatory cascade is set in motion by minor alterations in the endothelium, which are subsequently amplified in sequential steps (Fig. 2.3). These culminate in outright tissue destruction.

Table 2.4. Integrins[59,63,65]

Integrin	α β chain	Distribution	Ligand	Comment
VLA 1-6 (very late antigen)	α 1-6 / β1 (CD49 a-f / CD29)	Leukocytes, platelets, smooth muscle cells	Laminin, collagen, fibronectin, VCAM1	VLA4-VCAM1 pair involved in Peyer's patch homing
LFA 1 (leukocyte-associated antigen)	α 1 / β2 (CD11a/CD18)	All leukocytes	ICAM 1, 2, 3	Constitutive expression; role in strong adhesion
MAC 1 (macrophage antigen complex)	α m / β2 (CD11b/CD18)	Myeloid cells	iC3b (complement system)	Phagocytosis of microorganisms coated with iC3b
p150, 95	α x / β2 (CD11c/CD18)	Myeloid cells	iC3b (complement system)	Phagocytosis of microorganisms coated with iC3b

Table 2.5. Immunoglobulin supergene family[59, 62-65]

Immunoglobulin supergene family member	Distribution	Ligand	Comment
ICAM 1 (CD54), **ICAM 2** (intercellular adhesion molecule)	Endothelial cells, leukocytes	LFA 1	Small amounts on resting cells. Marked up-regulated during inflammation or antigen recognition.
LFA 2 (CD2) (lymphocyte function-associated antigen)	Thymocytes, T cells, NK cells	LFA 3, CD48, CD59	Role in signal transduction and activation of lymphoid cells
LFA3 (CD58)	All human cells except thymocytes	LFA 2	
VCAM 1 (CD106) (vascular adhesion molecule)	Endothelial cells	VLA 4	Expression increased by inflammation. Role in Peyer's patch homing
PECAM 1 (CD31) (platelet/endothelial cell adhesion molecule)	Endothelial and platelet intercellular junctions	?	May play a role in thrombosis
CD4	T-cell subpopulation	MHC II	T-cell (T helper/inducer phenotype) activation
CD8	T-cell subpopulation	MHC I	T-cell (T suppressor/cytotoxic phenotype) activation
MHC II (major histo-compatibility antigen)	Activated T, B and endothelial cells, monocytes	CD4	Presents peptides derived by endocytosis
MHC I	All nucleated cells	CD8	Presents endogenous, synthesized (viral) antigens
TCR (T-cell receptor)	T cells	MHC I or II	T-cell antigen recognition activation and proliferation
CD3	Complexed to TCR in all T cells	none	T-cell activation and proliferation

The inflammatory cascade is set in motion by endothelial activation as a result of ischemia, surgical manipulation or allorecognition. Platelet activating factor (PAF), which is not constitutively present in resting endothelial cells, appears on the cell surface,[63] and the activated endothelial cells begin to synthesize and secrete IL-8 and other cytokines.[56] Under the influence of these agents, selectins appear on the endothelial surface and vasodilatation occurs, causing circulating leukocytes to slow down.[61] Through serial interactions with these selectins, leukocytes come to a stop (Fig. 2.5a).[61,63-65] Leukocytes, now bound to endothelial selectins, come into contact with cytokines and activating surface endothelial molecules like PAF.[56,61] In response to these signals, leukocytes begin to synthesize and express their own surface adhesion molecules, the integrins (e.g, LFA-1). Similarly activated endothelial cells begin to express corresponding counter-receptors (e.g., ICAM-1). Interaction between these structures results in strong leukocyte binding to vasculature and further cell activation (Fig. 2.5b). While the leukocyte LFA-1 binds its endothelial counter-receptor, the cytoplasmic domain of the integrin molecules interacts with the cell's cytoskeleton, changing the leukocyte's motility and shape (Fig. 2.5c).[61] Through incompletely understood mechanisms, this allows coordinated adhesion and de-adhesion. As a result, leukocytes initiate diapedesis between endothelial cells. Once through the endothelial barrier, activated leukocytes breach the basement membrane by releasing degrading enzymes, and then begin migration into tissues.[56]

In addition to promoting antigen-independent inflammatory interactions, adhesion molecules also participate in antigen-dependent T-cell activation (Fig. 2.1). When the TCR comes into contact with its target antigen, an intercellular signal converts LFA-1 from a state of low avidity to one of high avidity.[12] LFA-1 then binds ICAM-1 on the APC surface. This stabilizes TCR binding to its target, facilitating antigen-dependent T-cell activation. After binding their corresponding ligands on the APC surface, LFA-1 and LFA-2 transduce a signal which synergizes with or augments activating signals from the TCR.[66-68] Thus adhesion molecules, like CD4, potentiate T-cell activation both by facilitating TCR contact with its target and by transmitting amplifying signals to the cytoplasm. Accordingly, preventing LFA-1 or LFA-2 interaction with their respective APC ligands interferes with T-cell activation.[69,70]

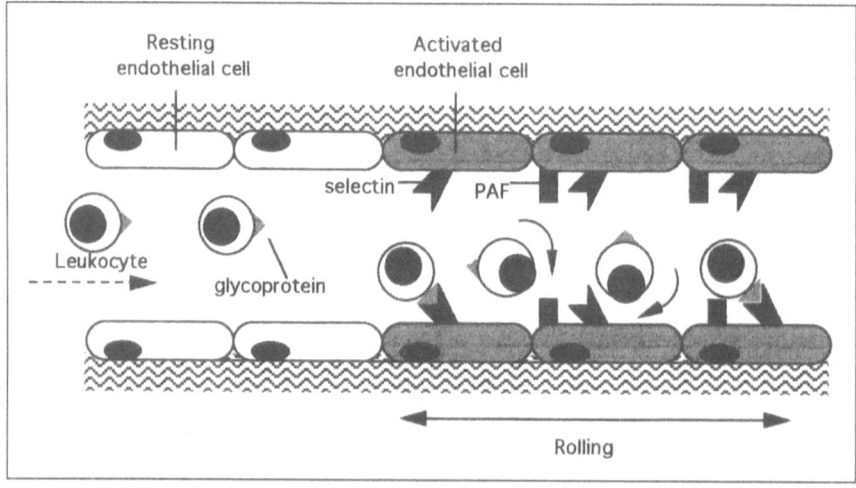

Fig. 2.5a. Initial contact. Activated endothelial cells express upregulated selectins and platelet activating factor (PAF). Repeated selectin binding brings circulating leukocytes to a stop. Neutrophils roll along the endothelium before stopping.

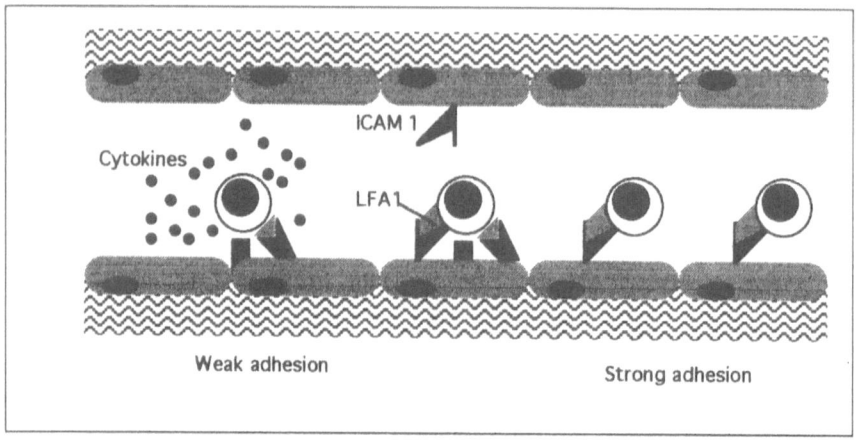

Fig. 2.5b. Adhesion to endothelium. Leukocytes bound to selectins are forced to stay in contact with PAF and in an area of high cytokine concentration. As a result, ICAM-1 and LFA-1 appear on endothelial and leukocyte surfaces, resulting in strong adhesions.

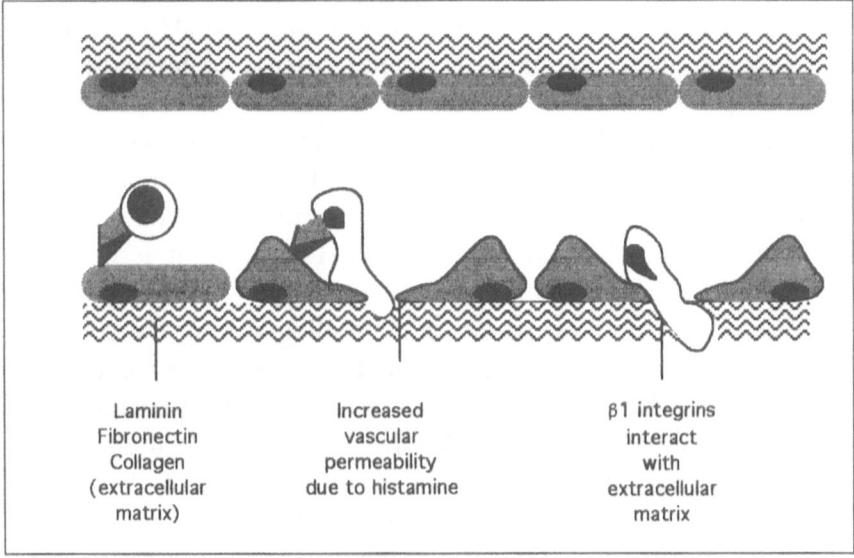

Fig. 2.5c. Migration into tissues. Integrin molecules cause changes in cytoskeleton, initiating diapedesis. Leukocytes then release enzymes which breach the basement membrane.

EXPERIMENTAL USE OF ANTI-ADHESION MONOCLONAL ANTIBODIES

Tolerance induction with monoclonal antibodies to adhesion molecules

Because of their crucial role in T-cell activation, adhesion molecules represent an attractive target for MoAb-based immunosuppression. In fact, MoAbs to adhesion molecules have been remarkably effective in some murine models. MoAbs to vascular adhesion molecule-1 (VCAM-1) have induced long-term murine cardiac allograft acceptance.[71] Similarly striking results have also been obtained with MoAb combinations targeting T cell and APC receptor-ligand pairs, such as LFA-1 and its ligand ICAM-1,[69] or LFA2 (CD2) and its ligand CD48.[70] With such therapy, the TCR presumably binds its target without concomitant adhesion molecule interactions, resulting in an incomplete activation signal. Under these circumstances, T cells specifically reactive with donor antigen may be rendered anergic instead of being sensitized.[41]

Nonhuman primate models of anti-adhesion monoclonal antibodies

The striking results observed in these rodent allograft models led to further preclinical studies in monkeys of BIRR1, an anti-ICAM-1 (CD54) MoAb.[72] The distribution of ICAM-1 expression in cynomolgus monkeys is similar to that of humans: both species express low levels of ICAM-1 on normal kidney endothelium; and during cellular rejection, both express increased concentrations of ICAM-1 on endothelial cells, infiltrating monocytes and tubular cells. Since BIRR1, a murine anti-human ICAM-1 MoAb, is crossreactive with cynomolgus ICAM-1 antigen, it is likely to have similar effects in both species.

Monkey allograft recipients of renal allografts mismatched for MHC I and II antigens were treated with a 12-day course of BIRR1. The MoAb was administered during the peritransplant period as the sole immunosuppressive agent (0.01-2 mg/kg/day). Allograft survival was significantly prolonged (24 ± 2.4 vs. 9.2 ± 0.6 days for controls; $p < 0.001$.) Biopsies during BIRR1 administration showed decreased T-cell infiltration and decreased arterial endothelial inflammation compared with controls. No BIRR1-induced changes were detected in circulating T cells. These results confirm that ICAM-1 plays a crucial role in the alloresponse and that targeting this molecule provides a substantial immunosuppressive effect.

Monoclonal antibodies in ischemic reperfusion injury

Reperfusion of devascularized tissues restores oxygen delivery, interrupting the cellular damage resulting from ischemia. Paradoxically, an additional ischemic injury occurs when circulation is reestablished. This reperfusion injury is mediated predominantly by neutrophils, and can be markedly attenuated by neutrophil depletion.[73] As noted earlier, ischemia activates endothelium, resulting in cytokine release and adhesion molecule upregulation. These signals cause circulating neutrophils to adhere to vascular endothelium and infiltrate the reperfused ischemic tissues. There, they release toxic proteases and reactive oxygen metabolites that damage the ischemic organ.[74]

In the cynomolgus model, a transient rise in serum creatinine is often detected during the first several days following renal transplantation. This spontaneously reversible dysfunction is the result of mild ischemic damage that occurs during kidney procurement.

Interestingly, clinical evidence for this acute tubular necrosis was markedly reduced in monkeys receiving the anti-ICAM-1 MoAb. This observation is supportive of the postulate that reperfusion of an ischemic organ leads to an inflammatory injury in which adhesion molecules play a crucial role, and has led to specific attempts to block this process with anti-adhesion molecule MoAbs. For instance, a MoAb to L-selectin (DREG-200) exerted a significant cardioprotective effect in a feline model of myocardial ischemia by attenuating neutrophil accumulation.[75] Similarly, MoAbs to ICAM-1 have provided a protective effect in animal models of kidney, heart, brain and liver reperfusion.[76-79]

CLINICAL TRIALS OF MONOCLONAL ANTIBODIES TO ADHESION MOLECULES

Despite the availability of effective organ preservation modalities, some degree of reperfusion injury invariably accompanies transplant procedures. Generally, this complication is reversible and manageable clinically. However, because adhesion molecules participate in antigen-specific interactions, their upregulation during reperfusion, although antigen-independent, could still potentiate rejection. For this reason, ischemic injury may affect not only early allograft function but also the intensity of the subsequent alloresponse, and therefore long-term graft survival. Clinical observations support this hypothesis. For example, living-unrelated donor renal transplantation may result in fewer rejection episodes and better long-term survival than cadaveric transplantation.[80] Similarly, a higher number of rejection episodes have been detected in cadaveric renal allografts with delayed function compared to those with good early function.[81] In fact, early renal function is one of the major determinants of eventual graft outcome.[81] Limiting preservation injury should therefore improve both early and late allograft survival. Thus, we and others have been particularly interested in the development of induction immunosuppressive regimens that incorporate the use of anti-adhesion molecule strategies.

Anti-ICAM-1

The encouraging background studies in nonhuman primates led to a phase I clinical study to evaluate the toxicity, dosage requirements and potential efficacy of BIRR1 in cadaver donor renal allograft recipients.[82] The initial trial selected patients at high risk for delayed graft function. Such patients included those receiving a second or greater allograft, those who were highly sensitized (PRA > 60%), and those receiving an allograft that was retrieved from an unstable donor or that had been preserved ex vivo for greater than 36 hours. As noted above, long-term (one-year) allograft survival is inferior in recipients with delayed graft function, generally being reported as approximately 65%, in contrast to the 80-85% survival rate observed in recipients with early allograft function.

Eighteen patients fulfilling the inclusion criteria were enrolled in the phase 1 trial. The initial protocol was designed to treat the patients with a BIRR1 dosage by weight comparable to the lowest dose found effective in the nonhuman primate studies. However, significant BIRR1 serum levels were not measurable in the first three patients, and all three suffered rejection episodes requiring OKT3 rescue. Subsequent patients were treated with increasing doses of BIRR1. Monitoring of serum MoAb levels indicated that there are considerably more CD54 combining sites available in dialyzed uremic patients than in the normal nonhuman primates previously studied. The protocol was therefore eventually modified to administer the entire 300-mg BIRR1 dosage over a 6-day interval.

With a follow-up of 24-36 months, 14 of the original 18 allografts in this trial (78%) continued with good to excellent function. This is encouraging in a recipient group preselected for relatively poor allograft prognosis. The fate of the contralateral kidneys from the same donors appears to confirm the high risk nature of these allograft. One of the contralateral kidneys was discarded by the recipient hospital because of the preservation history, and three others suffered primary nonfunction. This contrasts with 100% utilization of the donor kidneys and no instance of primary nonfunction in the 18 BIRR1-treated renal allograft recipients. Currently, overall allograft survival of the contralateral kidneys transplanted into conventionally treated patients is 50%. However, in interpreting these results, it is important to note that the contralateral kidneys were not randomly assigned and were generally transplanted at other institutions.

This initial clinical trial demonstrated that inhibition of leukocyte adhesion by BIRR1 therapy is well tolerated; and that it may be efficacious in controlling allograft rejection and possibly the severity of reperfusion injury. A randomized double-blind trial comparing BIRR1 to conventional induction therapy in cadaver donor renal allograft recipients has now enrolled over 180 patients at several U.S. transplant centers. A group of nonparticipating investigators recently reviewed the preliminary results, primarily to exclude evidence of unanticipated adverse events. They advised that enrollment of the originally targeted 200 patients be completed, and that a confirming trial be conducted in European transplant centers. Enrollment of patients into this second study has just been initiated.

Anti-LFA-1

LFA-1, the counter-receptor for ICAM-1 on leukocytes, has also been targeted for MoAb therapy. Bone marrow transplant patients were the first recipients of MoAb 25.3, which is directed against the CD11a epitope on LFA-1. This agent appeared to improve engraftment in a group of pediatric recipients that was compared to historical controls.[83] However, the same MoAb, administered to adult leukemic bone marrow recipients, was unable to prevent graft failure or rejection of T-cell-depleted HLA-matched transplants.[84] A MoAb directed against the CD18 epitope on LFA-1 was similarly ineffective.[85] In another study, a partial response to acute graft-versus-host disease (AGVHD) occurred in 80% of patients who received 25.3, but seven out of eight responding patients experienced a new episode of AGVHD.[86] Thus, anti-LFA-1 MoAb therapy has had only limited success in bone marrow transplantation.

In renal allograft recipients, 25.3 proved ineffective for the treatment of acute rejection.[87] Interestingly, patients developed little antibody response against this murine MoAb, suggesting a possible role for this agent in induction protocols. Accordingly, a pilot study was conducted in which 25.3 was administered to prevent rejection in renal allograft recipients. The MoAb was given daily for 10 days following transplantation, along with corticosteroids and azathioprine.[88] Cyclosporine was introduced on the ninth day. No clinical rejection occurred in the first month post-transplant. In the first three months, 42% of patients experienced an acute rejection episode which was completely reversible in all recipients. These results were comparable to those observed in a historical group of patients receiving ATG instead of the MoAb. The

MoAb administration was not associated with severe side-effects, although immunization to the MoAb was observed in 50% of patients. These encouraging results suggest that anti-LFA-1 therapy could be promising in preventing early rejection in kidney allograft recipients, and warrants continuing evaluation.

CONCLUSION

MoAbs targeting the CD4 antigen or other adhesion molecules provide the means for selective yet effective immunosuppression. As a result, clinical protocols incorporating these agents could reduce the morbidity of current regimens and possibly further improve allograft function. Even more interesting is the possibility of manipulating immunological events during the early stages of the alloresponse to induce allograft tolerance rather than sensitization to incompatibilities. This intriguing phenomenon has been achieved in numerous rodent models, utilizing brief courses of MoAbs targeting either the CD4 antigen or various adhesion molecules. These MoAbs apparently produce this common result by disabling the essential elements in the "second signal" required for T-cell activation. Unfortunately, these impressive results have not been reliably duplicated in nonrodent models to date. Current clinical protocols therefore continue to require long-term administration of conventional immunosuppressive agents. Nevertheless, MoAbs targeting the CD4 antigen or other adhesion molecules are being incorporated into induction therapy protocols with encouraging preliminary results. It seems likely that further experience with these agents will lead to the design of immunosuppressive protocols based on brief courses of sequentially administered MoAbs. These more complex strategies may be required to achieve true allograft tolerance, the ultimate goal of transplantation.

REFERENCES

1. Cosimi AB, Burton RC, Colvin RB et al. Treatment of acute renal allograft rejection with OKT3 monoclonal antibody. Transplantation 1981; 32:535-539.
2. Cosimi AB, Cho SI, Delmonico FL et al. A randomized clinical trial comparing OKT3 and steroids for treatment of hepatic allograft rejection. Transplant Proc 1987; 19:2431-2433.
3. Farges C, Samuel D, Bismuth H. Orthoclone OKT3 in liver transplantation. Transplantation Science 1992; 2:16-21.
4. Ortho Multicenter Transplant Study Group. A randomized clinical trial of OKT3 monoclonal antibody for acute rejection of cadaveric

renal transplants. N Engl J Med 1985; 313:337-342.

5. Ponticelli C, Rivolta E, Tarantino A et al. Treatment of severe rejection of kidney transplant with Orthoclone OKT3. Clin Transplantation 1987; 1:99-103.

6. Robbins RC, Oyer PE, Stinson EB et al. The use of monoclonal antibodies after heart transplantation. Transplant Sci 1992; 2:22-27.

7. Waid TH, Lucas BA, Thompson JS et al. Treatment of acute cellular rejection with T10B9.1A-31 or OKT3 in renal allograft recipients. Transplantation 1992; 53:80-86.

8. Frenken LA, Hoitsma AJ, Tax WJ et al. Prophylactic use of anti-CD3 monoclonal antibody WT32 in kidney transplantation. Transplant Proc 1991; 23:1072-1073.

9. Sablinski T, Hancock WW, Tilney NL et al. CD4 monoclonal antibodies in organ transplantation—a review of progress. Transplantation 1991; 52:579-589.

10. Auchincloss HJ, Sachs DH. Transplantation and graft rejection. In: Paul WE, ed. Fundamental Immunology. 3rd ed. New York:Raven Press, 1993:1099-1141.

11. Doyle C. Interaction between CD4 and class II MHC molecules mediates cell adhesion. Nature 1987; 330:256-259.

12. Springer TA. Adhesion receptors of the immune system. Nature 1990; 346:425-34.

13. Weiss A. T lymphocyte activation. In: Paul WE, ed. Fundamental Immunology. 3rd ed. New York:Raven Press, 1993:467-504.

14. Swain ST. T cell subsets and the recognition of MHC class. Immunol Rev 1983; 74:129-142.

15. Sprent J, Webb SR. Function and specificity of T cell subsets in the mouse. Adv Immunol 1987; 41:39-133.

16. Bishop DK, Shelby J, Eichwald EJ. Mobilization of T lymphocytes following cardiac transplantation. Evidence that CD4-positive cells are required for cytotoxic T lymphocyte activation, inflammatory endothelial development, graft infiltration, and acute allograft rejection. Transplantation 1992; 53:849-57.

17. Rosenberg AS, Munitz TI, Maniero TG et al. Cellular basis of skin allograft rejection across a class I major histocompatibility barrier in mice depleted of CD8+ T cells in vivo. J Exp Med 1991; 173:1463-1471.

18. Bishop DK, Chan S, Li W et al. CD4-positive helper T lymphocytes mediate mouse cardiac allograft rejection independent of donor alloantigen specific cytotoxic T lymphocytes. Transplantation 1993; 56:892-897.

19. Sayegh MH, Sablinski T, Tanaka K et al. Effects of BWH-4 anti-CD4 monoclonal antibody on rat vascularized cardiac allografts before and after engraftment. Transplantation 1991; 51:296-9.

20. Sablinski T, Sayegh MH, Kut JP et al. The importance of targeting the CD4+ T cell subset at the time of antigenic challenge for

induction of prolonged vascularized allograft survival. Transplantation 1992; 53:219-21.

21. Cosimi AB, Delmonico FL, Wright JK et al. Prolonged survival of nonhuman primate renal allograft recipients treated only with anti-CD4 monoclonal antibody. Surgery 1990; 108:406-13.

22. Greenwood J, Clark M, Waldmann H. Structural motifs involved in human IgG antibody effector functions. Eur J Immunol 1993; 23:1098-104.

23. Hancock WW, Sayegh MH, Sablinski T et al. Blocking of mononuclear cell accumulation, cytokine production, and endothelial activation within rat cardiac allografts by CD4 monoclonal antibody therapy. Transplantation 1992; 53:1276-80.

24. Shizuru JA, Seydel KB, Flavin TF et al. Induction of donor-specific unresponsiveness to cardiac allografts in rats by pretransplant anti-CD4 monoclonal antibody therapy. Transplantation 1990; 50:366-373.

25. Pearson TC, Bushell AR, Darby CR et al. Lymphocyte changes associated with prolongation of cardiac allograft survival in adult mice using anti-CD4 monoclonal antibody. Clin Exp Immunol 1993; 92:211-7.

26. Darby CR, Bushell A, Morris PJ et al. Nondepleting anti-CD4 antibodies in transplantation. Evidence that modulation is far less effective than prolonged CD4 blockade. Transplantation 1994; 57:1419-26.

27. Powelson JA, Knowles RW, Delmonico FL et al. CDR-grafted OKT4A monoclonal antibody in cynomolgus renal allograft recipients. Transplantation 1994; 57:788-93.

28. Horneff G, Emmrich F, Reiter C et al. Persistent depletion of CD4+ T cells and inversion of the CD4/CD8 T cell ratio induced by anti-CD4 therapy. J Rheumatol 1992; 19:1845-50.

29. Sprent J. T lymphocytes and the thymus. In: Paul WE, ed. Fundamental Immunology. 3rd ed. New York:Raven Press, 1993:75-109.

30. Kisielow P, Bluthmann H, Staerz UD et al. Tolerance in T-cell-receptor transgenic mice involves deletion of nonmature CD4+8+ thymocytes. Nature 1988; 333:742-6.

31. O'Toole CM, Maher P, Spiegelhalter DJ et al. 'Rejection or infection' predictive value of T-cell subject ratio, before and after heart transplantation. J Heart Transplant 1985; 4:518-24.

32. Shen SY, Weir MR, Kosenko A et al. Reevaluation of T cell subset monitoring in cyclosporine-treated renal allograft recipients. Transplantation 1985; 40:620-3.

33. Darby CR, Morris PJ, Wood KJ. Evidence that long-term cardiac allograft survival induced by anti- CD4 monoclonal antibody does not require depletion of CD4+ T cells. Transplantation 1992; 54:483-90.

34. Burkhardt K, Charlton B, Mandel TE. An increase in the survival

of murine H-2-mismatched cultured fetal pancreas allografts using depleting or nondepleting anti-CD4 monoclonal antibodies, and a further increase with the addition of cyclosporine. Transplantation 1989; 47:771-5.

35. Lehmann M, Sternkopf F, Metz F et al. Induction of long-term survival of rat skin allografts by a novel, highly efficient anti-CD4 monoclonal antibody. Transplantation 1992; 54:959-62.

36. Wee SL, Stroka DM, Preffer FI et al. The effects of OKT4A monoclonal antibody on cellular immunity of nonhuman primate renal allograft recipients. Transplantation 1992; 53:501-7.

37. Tite JP, Sloan A, Janeway CJ. The role of L3T4 in T cell activation:L3T4 may be both an Ia-binding protein and a receptor that transduces a negative signal. J Mol Cell Immunol 1986; 2:179-190.

38. Pearson TC, Madsen JC, Larsen CP et al. Induction of transplantation tolerance in adults using donor antigen and anti-CD4 monoclonal antibody. Transplantation 1992; 54:475-83.

39. Bushell A, Morris PJ, Wood KJ. Induction of operational tolerance by random blood transfusion combined with anti-CD4 antibody therapy. A protocol with significant clinical potential. Transplantation 1994; 58:133-9.

40. Qin SX, Wise M, Cobbold SP et al. Induction of tolerance in peripheral T cells with monoclonal antibodies. Eur J Immunol 1990; 20: 2737-2745.

41. Bretscher P. The two-signal model of lymphocyte activation twenty-one years later. Immunol Today 1993; 13:74-76.

42. Pearson TC, Hamano K, Morris PJ et al. Anti-CD4 monoclonal antibody-induced allograft survival is associated with a defect in interleukin-2-dependent T-cell activation. Transplant Proc 1993; 25:786-7.

43. Herbert J, Roser B. Strategies of monoclonal antibody therapy that induce permanent tolerance of organ transplants. Transplantation 1988; 46:128S-134S.

44. Alters SE, Song HK, Fathman CG. Evidence that clonal anergy is induced in thymic migrant cells after anti-CD4-mediated transplantation tolerance. Transplantation 1993; 56:633-8.

45. Heinrich G, Gram H, Kocher HP et al. Characterization of a human T cell-specific chimeric antibody (CD7) with human constant and mouse variable regions. J Immunol 1989; 143:3589-3597.

46. Riechmann L, Clark M, Waldmann H et al. Reshaping human antibodies for therapy. Nature 1988; 332:323-7.

47. Boulianne GL, Hozumi N, Shulman MJ. Production of functional chimaeric mouse/human antibody. Nature 1984; 312:643-6.

48. Delmonico FL, Cosimi AB, Kawai T et al. Non-human primate responses to murine and humanized OKT 4A. Transplantation 1993; 55:722-728.

49. Meiser BM, Reiter C, Reichenspurner H et al. Chimeric mono-clonal CD4 antibody—a novel immunosuppressant for clinical heart transplantation. Transplantation 1994; 58:419-23.
50. Horneff G, Burmester GR, Emmrich F et al. Treatment of rheu-matoid arthritis with an anti-CD4 monoclonal antibody. Arthritis Rheum 1991; 34:129-140.
51. Reinke P, Volk HD, Miller H et al. Anti-CD4 therapy of acute rejection in long-term renal allograft recipients [letter]. Lancet 1991; 338:702-3.
52. Morel P, Vincent C, Cordier G et al. Anti-CD4 monoclonal anti-body administration in renal transplanted patients. Clin Immunol Immunopathol 1990; 56:311-22.
53. Land W. Monoclonal antibodies in 1991:new potential options in clinical immunosuppressive therapy. Clin Transplantation 1991; 5: 493-500.
54. Tilney NL, Kupiec-Weglinski JW. The immunobiology of acute allograft rejection. In: Brent L, Sells RA, eds. Organ Transplanta-tion: Current Clinical and Immunological Concepts. London: Bailliere Tindall, 1989:19-38.
55. Grisham MB, Hernandez LA, Granger DN. Xanthine oxidase and neutrophil infiltration in intestinal ischemia. Am J Physiol 1986; 251:G567-G574.
56. Pober JS, Cotran RS. The role of endothelial cells in inflamma-tion. Transplantation 1990; 50:537-544.
57. Lasky LA. Selectins: interpreters of cell-specific carbohydrate infor-mation during inflammation. Science 1992; 258:964-969.
58. Mulligan MS, Paulson JC, De Frees S et al. Protective effects of oligosaccharides in P-selectin-dependent lung injury. Nature 1993; 364:149-51.
59. Azuma H, Heemann UW, Tullius SG et al. Cytokines and adhe-sion molecules in chronic rejection. Clin Transplant 1994; 8:168-80.
60. Gearing A, Newman W. Circulating adhesion molecules in disease. Immunol Today 1993; 14:506-512.
61. Heemann UW, Tullius SG, Azuma H et al. Adhesion molecules and transplantation. Ann Surg 1994; 219:4-12.
62. Shevach EM. Accessory molecules. In: Paul WE, ed. Fundamental Immunology. 3rd ed. New York: Raven Press, 1993:531-575.
63. Zimmerman GA, Prescott SM, McIntyre TM. Endothelial cell in-teractions with granulocytes: tethering and signaling molecules. Immunol Today 1992; 13:93-100.
64. Berg EL, McEvoy LM, Berlin C et al. L-selectin-mediated lym-phocyte rolling on MAdCAM-1 [see comments]. Nature 1993; 366:695-8.
65. Shimizu Y, Newman W, Tanaka Y et al. Lymphocyte interactions with endothelial cells. Immunol Today 1992; 13:106-12.
66. Kato K, Koyanagi M, Okada H et al. CD48 is a counter-receptor

for mouse CD2 and is involved in T cell activation. J Exp Med 1992; 176:1241-9.

67. Van Seventer G, Shimizu Y, Horgan KJ et al. The LFA-1 ligand ICAM-1 provides an important costimulatory signal for T cell receptor-mediated activation of resting T cells. J Immunol 1990; 144:4579-86.

68. Bierer BE, Sleckman BP, Ratnofsky SE et al. The biologic roles of CD2, CD4, and CD8 in T-cell activation. Annu Rev Immunol 1989; 7:579-99.

69. Isobe M, Yagita H, Okumura K et al. Specific acceptance of cardiac allograft after treatment with antibodies to ICAM-1 and LFA-1. Science 1992; 255:1125-7.

70. Qin L, Chavin KD, Lin J et al. Anti-CD2 receptor and anti-CD2 ligand (CD48) antibodies synergize to prolong allograft survival. J Exp Med 1994; 179:341-6.

71. Orosz CG, Ohye RG, Pelletier RP et al. Treatment with anti-vascular cell adhesion molecule 1 monoclonal antibody induces long-term murine cardiac allograft acceptance. Transplantation 1993; 56:453-60.

72. Cosimi AB, Conti D, Delmonico FL et al. In vivo effects of monoclonal antibody to ICAM-1 (CD54) in nonhuman primates with renal allografts. J Immunol 1990; 144:4604-4612.

73. Klausner JM, Anner H, Paterson IS et al. Lower torso ischemia-induced lung injury is leukocyte dependent. Ann Surg 1988; 208:761-7.

74. Entman ML, Michael L, Rossen RD et al. Inflammation in the course of early myocardial ischemia. Faseb J 1991; 5:2529-37.

75. Ma XL, Weyrich AS, Lefer DJ et al. Monoclonal antibody to L-selectin attenuates neutrophil accumulation and protects ischemic reperfused cat myocardium. Circulation 1993; 88:649-58.

76. Byrne JG, Smith WJ, Murphy MP et al. Complete prevention of myocardial stunning, contracture, low-reflow, and edema after heart transplantation by blocking neutrophil adhesion molecules during reperfusion. J Thorac Cardiovasc Surg 1992; 104:1589-96.

77. Clark WM, Madden KP, Rothlein R et al. Reduction of central nervous system ischemic injury by monoclonal antibody to intercellular adhesion molecule. J Neurosurg 1991; 75:623-7.

78. Kelly KJ, Williams WJ, Colvin RB et al. Antibody to intercellular adhesion molecule 1 protects the kidney. Proc Natl Acad Sci USA 1994; 91:812-6.

79. Suzuki S, Toledo PL. Monoclonal antibody to intercellular adhesion molecule 1 as an effective protection for liver ischemia and reperfusion injury. Transplant Proc 1993; 25:3325-7.

80. Terasaki PI, Cecka JM, Lim C et al. Overview. In: Terasaki PI, Cecka JM, eds. Clinical Transplants 1991. Los Angeles: UCLA Tissue Typing Laboratory, 1991:409-430.

81. Halloran PF, Aprile MA, Farewell V et al. Early function as the principal correlate of graft survival. Transplantation 1988; 46:223-8.

82. Haug CE, Colvin RB, Delmonico FL et al. A phase I trial of immunosuppression with anti-ICAM-1 (CD54) MoAb in renal allograft recipients. Transplantation 1993; 55:766-72.

83. Fischer A, Griscelli C, Blanche S et al. Prevention of graft failure by an anti-HLFA-1 monoclonal antibody in HLA-mismatched bone-marrow transplantation. Lancet 1986; 2:1058-61.

84. Maraninchi D, Mawas C, Stoppa AM et al. Anti LFA1 monoclonal antibody for the prevention of graft rejection after T cell-depleted HLA-matched bone marrow transplantation for leukemia in adults. Bone Marrow Transplant 1989; 4:147-50.

85. Baume D, Kuentz M, Pico JL et al. Failure of a CD18/anti-LFA1 monoclonal antibody infusion to prevent graft rejection in leukemic patients receiving T-depleted allogeneic bone marrow transplantation. Transplantation 1989; 47:472-4.

86. Stoppa AM, Maraninchi D, Blaise D et al. Anti-LFA1 monoclonal antibody (25.3) for treatment of steroid-resistant grade III-IV acute graft-versus-host disease. Transpl Int 1991; 4:3-7.

87. Le Mauff B, Hourmant M, Rougier JP et al. Effect of anti-LFA1 (CD11a) monoclonal antibodies in acute rejection in human kidney transplantation. Transplantation 1991; 52:291-296.

88. Hourmant M, Le Mauff B, Le Meur Y et al. Administration of an anti-CD11a monoclonal antibody in recipients of kidney transplantation. A pilot study. Transplantation 1994; 58:377-80.

CHAPTER 3

THE CLINICAL AND EXPERIMENTAL USE OF MONOCLONAL ANTIBODIES TO THE IL-2 RECEPTOR

Peter L. Amlot

INTRODUCTION

The immune system is economical with the number of antigen specific cells available to counter intermittent and infrequent antigenic challenges from infectious organisms and relies upon rapid cellular expansion in times of need. Cellular recognition of specific antigens leads to rapid proliferation of antigen specific cells and this process is called clonal expansion. Along with this clonal expansion there is also a diversification of potential effector cells and mechanisms. The response to antigen exposure is thus characterised by amplification. Initiating events in this amplification make appropriate targets for manipulating the immune system in a specific manner. Identification of interleukin 2 (IL-2) as an important T-cell growth factor[1] was followed by the development of a monoclonal antibody (MoAb), anti-Tac, recognizing the IL-2 receptor (IL-2R).[2] The early involvement of IL-2 in T-cell proliferation together with the acquisition of a MoAb that interfered with the function of IL-2 gave rise to hope that specific manipulation of the immune

Monoclonal Antibodies in Transplantation, edited by Lucienne Chatenoud. © 1995 R.G. Landes Company.

system was achievable. It has been said that the interaction between IL-2 and IL-2 receptors determines the magnitude and duration of the immune response. Either blocking of IL-2R or eliminating cells expressing IL-2R could be beneficial in suppressing
unwanted immune responses. Blocking clonal expansion would prevent production of sufficient cells to cause destructive immune responses while elimination of the antigen specific cells would lead directly to an antigen specific tolerance. Intervention at a stage preceding
amplification suggests that IL-2/IL-2R directed therapy was more likely
to be of prophylactic benefit than for reversing ongoing immune responses but does not exclude the latter.

   The hope of a purely selective manipulation of the immune
system was soon realized to be fanciful when the widespread effects of IL-2 were appreciated. IL-2 is the major proliferation-in-
ducing cytokine for mature T cells that also induces differentiation of cytotoxic T lymphocytes (CTL). At earlier stages IL-2 is
involved in the development of thymocytes and their expression
of the T-cell receptor (TCR).[3] IL-2 also affects the growth and
differentiation of B cells, monocytes and macrophages, epidermal
dendritic cells[4] as well as antigen-independent natural killer (NK)[5,6]
and lymphokine-activated killer (LAK) cells.[7,8] B cells can express
the IL-2R and IL-2 stimulation is associated with an increase in
IgM production as well as growth. IL-2 is even involved outside
the specific immune system via IL-2R mediated events in
myelopoiesis.[9] The many target cells and widespread effects of a
cytokine like IL-2 is called pleiotropy. A separate problem, revealed
by a deeper understanding of the IL-2/IL-2R system, is that of
redundancy. This means that more than one cytokine can carry
out the same function and therefore if one is blocked another can
replace it. This is a significant setback for the initially simple idea
that a MoAb to the IL-2R would specifically inhibit immune responses.

   This chapter will cover a number of issues related to the use
of MoAbs directed at the IL-2R and their use in transplantation.
First, our present understanding of the IL-2/IL-2R which has expanded rapidly over the last few years raises important questions
about how IL-2R directed therapy can work. Second, use of IL-2R
antibodies in both animals and clinical studies will be summarized
as well as their potential for inducing host tolerance to grafts. The
third issue relates to characteristics of MoAbs to the IL-2R re-

quired to make them effective and whether genetically engineered MoAbs will significantly augment their efficacy. Finally, an attempt will be made to predict future development of MoAb and other methods of targeting the IL-2R.

BIOLOGY OF THE IL-2/IL-2R SYSTEM

It became rapidly evident that the IL-2R molecule (55 kDa) defined by the MoAb anti-Tac[10] could not form the whole receptor. IL-2 cross-linking studies defined low, intermediate and high affinity binding sites on lymphocytes and the 55 kDa molecule was only involved in the low and high affinity receptors because anti-Tac could inhibit these but not the intermediate affinity receptor. In addition, large granular lymphocytes (LGL) and NK cells could respond to IL-2 but they did not express the 55 kDa molecule. Co-precipitation of proteins cross-linked by IL-2 led to the discovery of a 75 kDa molecule as a second chain in the IL-2R but still the experimental data did not fit with a two-chain receptor. The 75 kDa chain expressed by LGL or transfected into lymphoid cells, not expressing the 55 kDa chain, had intermediate affinity IL-2 binding sites. Certain non-lymphoid cells transfected with the 75 kDa chain were unable to bind IL-2[11] and also purified 75 kDa chains had only minimal IL-2 binding capability.[12] Furthermore fibroblasts transfected with both 55 and 75 kDa chains formed IL-2 binding sites with affinity higher than intermediate yet were unable to internalize IL-2 or deliver a signal that suggested the absence of a necessary subunit.[13] Lastly the number of 75 kDa molecules expressed by lymphoid cells was disproportionate to the number of intermediate affinity IL-2 binding sites because following exposure to IL-2 there was a 3-fold rise in 75 kDa chains without a corresponding rise in intermediate affinity binding sites.[14,15] All these observations meant that the 75 kDa molecule could not alone form an intermediate affinity binding site and it was known that the 55 kDa molecule did not contribute to it. Most recently a 64 kDa chain has been identified as part of the IL-2R to make a three chain complex.[16]

A diagram of the IL-2R complex is shown in Figure 3.1 and characteristics of the components within the IL-2/IL-2R system are given in Table 3.1. The structure and function of IL-2 is well conserved from mouse to man.[17] It is a core type glycoprotein composed of 133 amino acids and 10% carbohydrate making a

15 kDa sized molecule. A large proportion of the amino acids are
hydrophobic, a common feature of proteins interacting with cell
membrane receptors. There is evidence that IL-2 binds mono-
merically and monovalently to the 55 kDa chain.[18,19]

The 55 kDa molecule has been called the α chain (IL-2Rα)
and also CD25. The extracellular part of the chain is 219 amino
acids long with only 19 amino acids crossing the membrane and
13 amino acids in the cytoplasm. This cytoplasmic tail is too short
to transduce signals across the membrane. IL-2Rα probably acts
to accelerate IL-2 binding and to stabilize interactions between IL-2
and the IL-2R by increasing its affinity which in the absence of
IL-2Rα is low compared to other cytokine receptors. The "on"
and "off" rate of IL-2 for the IL-2Rα is very rapid and is only
delayed by the presence of other IL-2R chains (Table 3.1). IL-2Rα
is not part of any known family of receptors unlike its two partners in the IL-2R complex. IL-2Rα is shed as a soluble form into
the blood and in large amounts during IL-2 therapy.[20]

The 75 kDa molecule has been called the β chain (IL-2Rβ)
and also CD122. Upon activation the IL-2Rβ is upregulated about
5-fold whereas IL-2Rα is upregulated about 100-fold if initially it
can be detected at all.[21,22] The extracellular part of the β chain is
214 amino acids long with a 25 amino acid transmembrane portion

Table 3.1. Characteristics of IL-2R α, β and γ chains

Subunit	IL-2 affinity [A]	T$_{1/2}$ K$_d$ (min)	Internalization	Signal	Chromosome locus
α	+	0.5	–	–	**10** p14-15
β	±	1.6	–	–	**22** q11.2-12 [B]
γ	–	–	–	–	**X** q13 [C]
αβ	+++	18.5	± [D]	– [E]	
βγ	++	255.0	+	+	
αβγ	++++	255.0	+	+	

[A] Scale of affinity in Kd assessed in transfected fibroblasts:

–	negative		2+	intermediate	~1 nM
±	equivocal	100 nM	3+	pseudo-high	~100 pM
+	low	~10 nM	4+	high	~10 pM

αγ chains co-expressed = α alone. IL-2 is encoded on chromosome 4.
[B] Locus for several lymphoid neoplasms[137,138]
[C] Locus for X-SCID
[D] Disagreement between different groups
[E] Mutant cells lacking γ chain.[139]

and a 286 amino acid cytoplasmic tail. The cytoplasmic tail is long enough to transduce signals across the membrane but does not have any direct enzyme activity. It contains serine-rich and acidic-rich regions which are important for its signaling function (Fig. 3.1). The IL-2Rβ belongs to a new family of receptors known as the hematopoietin (or cytokine Type I) receptor superfamily

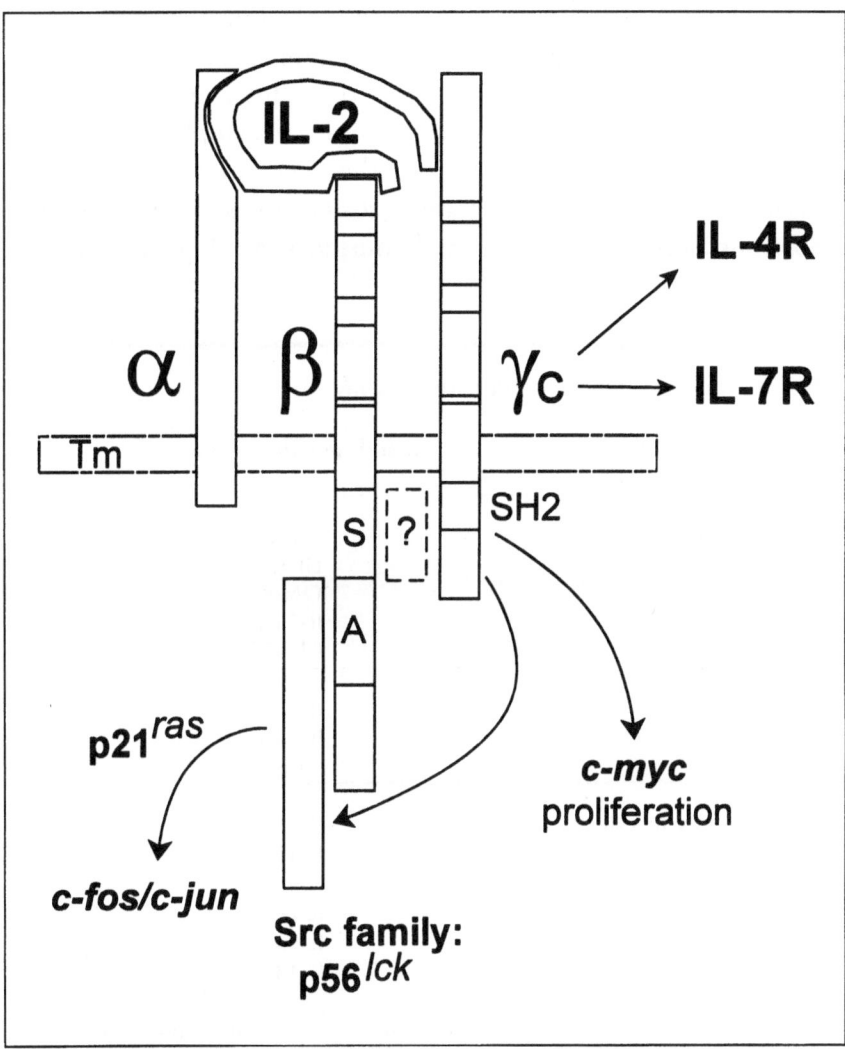

Fig. 3.1 IL-2/IL-2R binding and signaling.

▭	*Conserved cysteine residues*
▨	*WSXWS motif*
S	*Serine-rich region of IL-2Rβ*
A	*Acidic-rich region of IL-2Rβ*
?	*JAK-3 kinase?*

(Table 3.2). Most members of the haematopoietin receptor superfamily have two chains α and β with short and long cytoplasmic
tails respectively. The IL-2Rβ is also part of the receptor complex
for IL-15 and IL-T. It is probable that IL-T is identical to IL-15.
They both cause T-cell proliferation via the IL-2Rβ without interacting with the IL-2Rα and have equivalent molecular sizes of
14-15 kDa.[23-25]

The 64 kDa molecule is the IL-2Rγ chain but will be referred
to as γc because it is a chain common to a number of hematopoietin
receptors (Table 3.2). There are 232 extracellular amino acids in
its mature form, 28 transmembrane and 86 cytoplasmic amino
acids. Like IL-2Rβ, the γc belongs to the haematopoietin receptor
superfamily and does not contain tyrosine kinase activity in its
cytoplasmic domain.[26] Human and murine γc are highly homolo-

Table 3.2. Hematopoietin receptor superfamily

Signal transducer: common chain	Ligand-specific receptor
gp130	IL-6R
	LIF-R
	OM-R
	IL-11R
	CNTF-R
βc	IL-3Rα
	IL-5Rα
	GM-CSF-R
γc + IL-2Rβ	IL-2Rα
	IL-15R
γc	IL-4R
	IL-7R
	IL-9R
	IL-13R

LIF: leukemia inhibitory factor; OM: oncostatin M; CNTF: ciliary neurotrophic
factor; GM-CSF: granulocyte-macrophage colony stimulating factor;
βc: common β chain.
The family is homologous in the extracellular domains with conserved cysteine
residues and a perimembranous WSXWS motif. In the cytoplasm there is
homology of the SH2 region probably interacting with the same set of proteins
involved in signal transduction.[59,140] Single chain members of the family are
erythropoietin, growth hormone, prolactin and G-CSF receptors.

gous (70% identity) allowing the human β chain to function with murine γ_c. The γ_c is essential for internalization and signaling via IL-2. The γ_c is common to the IL-4,[27,28] IL-7[29,30] and possibly the IL-9 and IL-13 receptors. The γ_c increases binding affinity in all three systems: IL-2R by 70-fold, IL-4R by 2- to 3-fold and IL-7R by 5- to 10-fold. The association of γ_c with IL-4R may explain the observations that IL-4 inhibits IL-2 binding to some cell lines and down regulates the IL-2R.[31-33] IL-4 can inhibit IL-2 mediated growth[34,35] and a dose dependent inhibition or enhancement of IL-2 mediated generation of LAK cells.[36] IL-7 is a cofactor for TCR gene rearrangement in thymocytes[37] and a growth factor for thymocytes[38-40] and T cells.[41-45] The γ_c chain is located at the same site on chromosome Xq13 as X-linked severe combined immunodeficiency (X-SCID) and in X-SCID a variety of mutations of the γ_c chain have been described that render it nonfunctional.[46]

The extracellular domains of IL-2Rβ and γ_c chains provide the means by which IL-2 or IL-15 induces heterodimerisation of the cytoplasmic portions of the two chains. Homodimerisation is ineffective for signaling whereas heterodimerisation is sufficient and necessary. The IL-2/IL-2R interaction does not induce increased $[Ca^{2+}]_i$, phosphatidylinositol hydrolysis or protein kinase C activation but does induce tyrosine protein kinase activity similar to activation in other cytokine systems.[47] Three critical parameters leading to IL-2/IL-2R induced entry of T cells into proliferative cycle were defined as IL-2R density, IL-2 concentration and the duration of the interaction between the two.[48] In terms of the IL-2R chains, this correlates with rapid trapping of any extracellular IL-2 by IL-2Rα onto the cell membrane and in the presence of IL-2Rβ and γ_c retention of the IL-2 sufficiently long for internalization, signaling and activation to occur. IL-2 induces rapid tyrosine kinase activity with phosphorylation of many proteins including the IL-2Rβ. This is due to interaction between the acidic-rich region of the IL-2Rβ cytoplasmic tail and NH-terminal half of p56*lck* which is part of the Src family of tyrosine kinases. In different cell lineages (not containing p56*lck*) other family members (e.g. p59*fyn* or p53/56*lyn*) may be activated in an analogous manner. IL-2-induced tyrosine kinase activity is associated with p21*ras* linked to the activation of the nuclear oncogenes, *c-jun* and *c-fos* (Fig. 3.1). The 'serine-rich' region of the IL-2Rβ is important for induction of the *c-myc* gene and transit through the cell cycle.[49] This suggests a bifurcation in the signaling pathways similar to that seen with CSF-1.[50] IL-2 binding to the high affinity IL-2Rαβγ complex (Table 3.1) leads to stimulation of a number of catalytic molecules including protein tyrosine kinases, JAK 3 kinase, Raf-1 kinase, p21^{ras}, PI-3 kinase and proto-oncogenes.

Pleiotropy and redundancy characterize the cytokine system. For example IL-2, IL-4, IL-5, IL-6 and γ-IFN can all induce antibody production by B cells. IL-2, IL-4, IL-6 or leukemia inhibitory factor (LIF) gene disrupted ("knockout") mice have near normal development of T cells and only minor deficiencies of immunoglobulin production or decreased growth[51-53] which indicates that the missing cytokine can be replaced by others. Although early T cell development is normal in IL-2 "knockout" mice, half develop splenomegaly, lymphadenopathy and anaemia and die by 9 weeks while the remainder become ill with an autoimmune-like ulcerative colitis.[54] Mature T cells can develop in a SCID patient in the absence of IL-2 production.[55] A major problem in understanding signaling pathways may lie in the promiscuity of cytokine interactions within the hematopoietin receptor superfamily. Different chains may co-associate and be able to respond to other cytokines than those with which they normally associate. Disparity between cytokine deficiency and overexpression indicates compensatory (redundant) mechanisms in deficiency which contrasts with the severe disease seen in overexpression. Transgenic mice overexpressing IL-2 develop alopecia, skin infiltration and ataxia due to cerebellar infiltration by T cells;[56,57] overexpression of IL-6 produces severe defects (myeloma, mesangial proliferative glomerulonephritis) and LIF leads to cachexia, bone abnormalities, pancreatitis and thymic atrophy.

Multi-chain receptors of the hematopoietin receptor superfamily use a private ligand-specific receptor which confers specificity and shares a public class-specific signal transducer explaining why cytoplasmic signaling events are common to many cytokines (Table 3.2). There are many overlapping roles for the various ligand-specific receptors with the γc being shared among at least three and probably five while the IL-2Rβ chain is probably involved in at least two different receptors. The absence or nonfunction of the γc chain has a much more severe effect on the immune system because it leads to the inactivation of at least three cytokine systems (IL-2, IL-4, IL-7) for which compensation cannot be made in contrast to the loss of a single cytokine. A further overlap is seen with the IL-2Rβ chain which can induce T-cell proliferation not only through IL-2 but also IL-15/IL-T. In addition, GM-CSF is not only structurally related to IL-2[58,59] but has been shown capable of competing with IL-2 for the IL-2R complex.[60]

For MoAb therapy, the implications of these biological features of the IL-2/IL-2R system are important. First, single antibody MoAb therapy aiming to block interaction between IL-2 and IL-2R leaves several pathways available that can bypass its blockade, whereas strategies aimed at eliminating IL-2R⁺ cells would be more likely to succeed. Second, because the IL-2Rα has no signaling function, ligation by antibody should not lead to the cytokine release phenomena associated with CD3 or TCR MoAb therapy. Third, the bifurcation in signaling within the IL-2/IL-2R system may be exploitable for the purpose of immune modulation.

CELLULAR DISTRIBUTION OF IL-2R CHAINS

IL-2 is known to be involved in thymocyte proliferation and maturation and in the thymus IL-2Rα is expressed on CD4⁻CD8⁻ thymocytes (double negative) while IL-2Rβ is expressed on CD4⁺CD8⁺ (double positive) as well as thymocytes expressing TCRγδ. The γ_c is present on all thymocytes.[61] It is particularly relevant that double negative thymocytes express the conventional IL-7R[62] suggesting that IL-7 may be more important for thymocyte proliferation than IL-2. This interpretation is supported by the normal thymic development of IL-2 "knockout" mice compared to the thymic atrophy arising in mice treated with antibodies to IL-7 or IL-7R[62,63] and IL-7 is the only cytokine known to induce V(D)J rearrangement of the TCRβ chain.[37] IL-2 and IL-7 appear to control different stages of thymocyte differentiation. TCRγδ cells appear more dependent on IL-2 because they disappeared completely in IL-2 "knockout" mice.[54]

The expression of IL-2Rs on blood leukocytes is shown in Table 3.3. T-cell expression of the IL-2Rα at low levels is found in 10% of cord blood, 20% of adult blood and 20% of lymph nodes rising to 35% or higher in activated lymph node TCRαβ cells.[64] Most blood TCRγδ cells express IL-2Rα and TCRαβ cells bearing the "activated" isoform of the leukocyte common antigen, CD45RO, express IL-2Rα more frequently than those bearing the CD45RA isoform (40% compared to 5%).[64] These are in vivo equivalents of recently activated cells in vitro. IL-2Rβ is expressed constitutively by CD8+ cytotoxic cells.[14] The recent availability of MoAbs to the γ_c has revealed the very widespread expression of this receptor chain on all leukocytes and not merely mononuclear cells (Table 3.3).

Induction of both IL-2Rα and IL-2Rβ chains occurs rapidly on T cells, B cells and monocytes after stimulation with mitogens, anti-IgM and lipopolysaccharide (LPS) respectively. IL-2Rβ is increased on CD4 and CD8 cells in renal allograft rejection.[65]

IL-2Rβ chain appears more gradually on monocytes with 40% positive after 2 days. γ_c is either already present or appears almost immediately upon stimulation.[66]

Expression of IL-2Rβ is upregulated on mononuclear cells expressing the IL-2Rα chain as well as those not expressing it. Unexpectedly IL-2Rβ was found on embryonic fibroblasts and they may respond to IL-2 in the absence of γ_c.[67] IL-2Rβ is also expressed on epidermal dendritic cells.[68]

The distribution of IL-2R chains indicate that IL-2Rα is still the most restricted and selective for activated T cells, with more widespread expression of IL-2Rβ and extremely widespread expression of γ_c befitting its role as a common chain in a number of cytokine systems. MoAb therapy directed at γ_c seems impractical and even the use of therapy directed at the IL-2Rβ would lose some of the selectivity originally envisaged with IL-2Rα therapy.

Table 3.3. Leukocyte expression of IL-2R chains [A]

Cell lineage	% of blood cells expressing:		
	IL-2Rα	IL-2Rβ	γ_c
CD4	30	30	100
CD8	5	50	100
B cells	40	–	100
NK cells	–	90	90
Monocytes	–	10	70
Granulocytes	–	– [B]	80

[A] Results compiled from references[64,66,141-142]
[B] Granulocytes were found positive in one study[143] but not confirmed in a separate study.[66]

ANIMAL STUDIES ON THE EFFECT OF CD25 (IL-2Rα) MoAB THERAPY

CD25 MoAb therapy can prolong survival of heart, kidney, pancreas, small bowel and neural grafts in mice and rats[69] and of heart and kidney grafts in primates using CD25 MoAbs raised against human but cross-reacting with primate IL-2Rα. The histocompatibility barrier across which CD25 MoAb therapy can work varies according to the tissue transplanted and the MoAb used. Prolongation of murine heart graft survival was effective in two separate, fully allogeneic H_2 mismatches (Table 3.4) while for prevention of murine graft versus host disease (GVHD) it could only be achieved across minor histocompatibility barriers or in local GVHD using restricted numbers of donor T cells to initiate GVHD. CD25 MoAb therapy could neither prevent systemic GVHD in mice nor full-blown fatal GVHD in any animal model nor could it prolong skin graft survival unless combined with

Table 3.4. CD25 MoAb therapy in animal transplantation

Animal	Organ	MoAb	Effects of CD25 MoAb:		CsA synergy	Reference
			IL-2 block [A]	Prolongs GS [B]		
Mouse	Heart	M7/20	Yes	Yes		76
	GVHD	M7/20	Yes	Yes [C]		144
	GVHD	AMT-13	Yes	Yes [C]		145
Rat	Heart	ART-18	Yes	Yes	Yes	77,78
		ART-65	No	Slight		
		OX-39	Yes	No		
	Heart 2°	ART-18	Yes	Yes	Yes	146
Rat	Kidney	ART-18	Yes	Yes	Yes [D]	147
	Kidney	NDS 61	Yes	Yes [E]	Yes	70,71
Rat	Islets	ART-18	Yes	Yes	Yes	148
Monkey	Kidney	1-HT4-4H3	Yes	No		72
	Kidney	anti-Tac	Yes	Yes	No	72
	Heart	anti-Tac	Yes	Yes		73
	Kidney	Campath-6	Yes	Yes		74

[A] Blocks IL-2 binding to the IL-2R
[B] Graft survival usually doubled compared to controls
[C] Decreased GVHD towards minor MHC antigens[144] or in local GVHD.[145]
[D] A proportion of grafts survive indefinitely with a combination of ART-18 and ART-65.
[E] 67% of grafts survive indefinitely

X-irradiation. Most of the rat heart and kidney graft studies shown in Table 3.4 were across a semi-allogeneic RT1 barrier of F1 hybrid (Lew x BN) into parental strain (Lew). The exceptions were fully allogeneic RT1 heart and kidney transplants using the MoAb NDS 61.[70,71] The primate kidney and heart grafts were from outbred monkeys.[72-74] In virtually all of these animal models the outcome of CD25 MoAb therapy was a doubling of graft survival which rarely led to indefinite survival unless it was combined with other immunosuppressive therapy. The exception to this was NDS 61. Furthermore, CD25 MoAb therapy was almost always given as prophylaxis and for theoretical reasons it does not lend itself to reversal of established graft rejection. Where reversal of graft rejection has been achieved it was under specialized conditions not normally relevant for clinical use.[75]

The mechanism by which CD25 MoAb therapy prolonged graft survival was the object of several animal studies. The main areas of investigation concerned blocking IL-2 binding to its receptor and the elimination of IL-2Rα^+ cells. All effective CD25 MoAbs

Table 3.5. Characteristics of mouse anti-rat CD25 MoAbs

MoAb	Isotype	Epitope group	Affinity Kd (nM)	Sites/cell x 10³ [A]	↑GS [B]	Inhibition of IL-2 effects on:		
						MLR (%) [C]	IL-2R Binding	Growth
ART-18	IgG1	R1	1.9	75	Yes	50	Yes	Yes
NDS 61	IgG1	-	-	-	Yes	Yes	Yes	Yes
NDS63	IgG1	R1	-	-	Yes	Yes	Yes	Yes
NDS 66	IgG2a	R2	-	-	No	No	No	No
ART-65	IgG1	R2	1.2	28	Slight	14	No	No
ART-75	IgG2a	R2	1.8	165	No	14	No	No
ART-35	IgG1	R3	1.1	47	No	0	No	No
OX 39	IgG1	R4	0.8	61	No	25	Yes	No

[A] Glycosylated epitopes may explain the differences in number of binding sites per cell.
[B] Prolongs graft survival.
[C] % inhibition of the mixed lymphocyte reaction (MLR) in the presence of the MoAb.

blocked IL-2 binding to the IL-2Rα (Table 3.4) and also interfered with IL-2-driven proliferation (Table 3.5). CD25 MoAbs that bound to epitopes on the IL-2Rα that were not involved in IL-2 function were of no value unless they had an unusually strong lytic capability. Synergy of CD25 MoAbs with cyclosporine A (CsA) was found in many of the studies. Synergy in these cases was not formally tested but meant increased activity in the presence of sub-therapeutic doses of CsA. In only one study was pharmacologically-defined synergy truly found to occur.[70] There was general agreement that CsA augmented the effects of CD25 MoAb therapy in mice and rats but this was not seen with kidney transplants in cynomologous monkeys.[72] The ineffectiveness of CD25 MoAbs that did not interfere with IL-2-mediated function and synergy of effective CD25 MoAbs with CsA both pointed to an IL-2 blockade as an important component of their action.

Elimination of IL-2Rα⁺ cells was more difficult to establish. Evidence was found for depletion of IL-2Rα⁺ cells contributing to the action of some MoAbs[76,77] but not others.[70] Survival of heart grafts was not prolonged when rats were treated with Fab′ or F(ab′)₂ fragments of the CD25 MoAb (ART-18) despite their ability to block IL-2 binding and inhibit the MLR. IL-2R⁺ cells were present in the graft infiltrate of Fab′ and F(ab′)₂ treated rats but not with whole IgG ART-18. These features suggested that the Fc portion of the antibody was necessary to mediate antibody-dependent cellular cytotoxicity (ADCC) and lead to the elimination of IL-2Ra⁺ cells. In accord with these findings, graft survival rose in relation to the efficacy in ADCC of the ART-18 isotype switch variants: IgG2b > IgG1 > IgG2a.[78] However, an effective CD25 MoAb, NDS 63, was reported as being non-depleting.[79]

There were a number of other observations regarding effects of CD25 MoAb therapy in rats treated with ART-18 that did not apply to the main issues of IL-2 blockade and depletion of IL-2Rα⁺ cells but reveal some of the phenomenology of CD25 MoAb therapy. Both thymectomy and treatment with γ-IFN concurrently with ART-18 abrogated its beneficial effect on heart graft survival in rats.[69,78] These were interpreted as selective effects on suppressor cells and Th1 cells respectively but are difficult to interpret properly. Although kidney graft survival was prolonged by ART-18 therapy, kidney function remained poor throughout and IL-2Rα⁺ cells were not eliminated in kidney grafts unlike the findings in heart grafts.[80] IL-2Rα⁺ cells were more easily detected using the CD25 MoAb, OX 39, which detects a different epitope to ART-18 (Table 3.5) and this suggests that the cells were coated with ART-18 in vivo. Lastly, cellular infiltrates were not decreased in grafts during CD25 MoAb therapy, indeed CD8⁺ cells were increased compared with controls. Many of these phenomena were interpreted in terms of suppressor cell phenomena prevalent at the time. Today we would have to consider the possibility that CD8⁺ cells that express both IL-2Rβ and γ_c chains (Table 3.3) should not be responsive to CD25 MoAb therapy and the differences between heart and kidney grafts may relate to the amount of MHC Class I and II alloantigen expressed and hence their immunogenicity.

With most CD25 MoAbs and all graft types survival time was only doubled and the grafts were eventually lost. One reason has just been discussed and it will be of great interest to see when and if expression of mRNA for IL-7 and IL-15 appears in rejecting grafts normally and in the face of CD25 MoAb therapy. However, another contributory factor to graft loss was the development of rat or monkey anti-MoAb responses (AMA) which cleared the xenogeneic CD25 MoAbs from the circulation and neutralized their activity. Because of the homology between rat and mouse and human and primate immunoglobulin AMA responses are widely thought to be of little importance but rat AMA occurred within 10-14 days and graft loss occurred shortly afterwards. Similarly primates treated with murine anti-Tac developed AMA responses shortly before grafts were lost and in both species the AMA responses contained a high proportion of anti-idiotype antibodies. CsA inhibits the development of AMA and this must be considered another means by which "synergy" occurs with CD25 MoAb therapy.

There were marked differences in the therapeutic efficacy between different CD25 MoAbs. The fact that all effective MoAbs blocked IL-2 function suggested that this must form part of the role that CD25 MoAbs play in vivo. There was no direct effect of MoAb affinity on function unless the antibody recognized the IL-2 binding site on the IL-2R (Table 3.5). An interesting MoAb in this respect is OX 39 which may have a counterpart in 1-HT4-4H3 reacting with human IL-2Rα (Table 3.4). OX 39 was capable of blocking IL-2 binding to the IL-2R but had no effect on graft survival. Unlike other effective CD25 MoAbs, OX 39 was not efficient at blocking IL-2 driven proliferation[81] and it was found to be 10-20 times less efficient at blocking IL-2 binding to the high affinity (K_I = 10 M) than to the low affinity (K_I = 0.5 nM) IL-2R.[82] This suggests that the site to which OX 39 binds may be partly concealed by the assembly of IL-2R$\alpha\beta\gamma$ chains in the high affinity receptor compared to the easier accessibility of free IL-2Rα (low affinity receptor). Therefore selection of effective CD25 MoAbs has to consider not only IL-2 blockade but also functional inhibition of IL-2 which implies an ability to bind effectively to the high affinity IL-2R. This is a small proportion of the IL-2R for only 2-5% of IL-2R can bind at high affinity.[82] Lastly the CD25 MoAb, NDS 61 had a superiority over ART-18 for which there is no obvious explanation. It is likely that this resides once again in the fine binding site specificity of NDS 61 since it binds to the same epitope group as ART-18 and it has the same immunoglobulin isotype, IgG1, which means it should have no superior effector function. We will see that the same heterogeneity is apparent in CD25 MoAbs binding to human IL-2Rα.

Some lessons could be learned from animal studies regarding dosage. Optimal doses were usually in the range 0.2-0.3 mg/kg/day for 10 days. This translates to a dose of 15-20 mg in a 70 kg human. Doses used in primates are shown in the legend to Table 3.4 and were relatively high, translating to a dose of 70-140 mg in 70 kg human. However, in primates careful dose finding studies were not done and the best results were achieved at 0.05 mg/kg with anti-Tac which were probably attributed to chance.[72] The duration of CD25 MoAb therapy had to be greater than 3 days and no improvement was seen when given for longer than 10 days,[71,75] but this was probably determined by the rat AMA response arising by then and abolishing the effect of further MoAb therapy. Most of the therapies started at the time of transplantation but in primate studies were started 1- 2 days after grafting. In one rat study therapy started at day 5 or intermittently (days 5-9 and 15-19) achieved as good results as from the day of transplantation. One experiment using continuous infusion found the results less effective than the standard bolus injections.[75] It was also relevant that no adverse effects were reported with the administration of CD25 MoAbs which confirmed that no cytokine release was to be expected.

TOLERANCE INDUCTION

The holy grail in transplantation immunology is the induction of tolerance or anergy in the host towards allogeneic grafted tissue by means of a short course of immunomodulatory therapy. There are many studies which indicate that a relative deficiency of IL-2 can lead to tolerance. One model of transplantation tolerance involves exposing neonatal mice to semi-allogeneic cells or foreign soluble antigens which induce long term non-responsiveness to the specific antigen used during the neonatal period. Since neonatal tolerance can be reversed by administration of IL-2, it has been inferred that neonatal tolerance develops because there is a relative deficiency of IL-2 production early in life.[83-85] The relative deficiency in IL-2 production occurs also in several adult models of transplantation tolerance. Relatively small doses of IL-2 administered with large doses of *Mycobacterium bovis* to mice, rats and guinea pigs reverse the tolerance that normally develops towards *M. bovis*.[86] Indeed the establishment of tolerance may be related to its ability to suppress IL-2 production. Blood transfusion tolerised rats have a lower T cell expression of IL-2Rα and IL-2Rβ, low affinity IL-2Rs and at the time of their maximum responsiveness (day 3) they do not make IL-2.[87] TCR engagement in the absence of a co-stimulatory signal leads to unresponsiveness characterized by inability to produce IL-2.[88] Anergic T cells have been shown to have a defect in antigen-induced transcription of the IL-2 gene with down regulation of the transcription factor AP-1. Addition of IL-2 restores activity of the T cell and the AP-1 transcription factor.[89] CD4 MoAb induced clonal anergy to alloantigens in both CD4 and CD8 cells can be overcome by the addition of IL-2[90] and CD4 MoAb induced tolerance to a heart graft demonstrated a marked reduction in IL-2 RNA.[91] All of these tolerant or anergic states characterized by a deficient production of IL-2 are mimicked by cyclosporine (CsA) treatment but it is known that CsA does not normally induce tolerance and it can prevent tolerance developing in several models of autoimmune disease. IL-2 is not the only cytokine that can break the anergic state. Antigen or alloantigen presented to the TCR in the absence of costimulatory signals leads to anergy but in the presence of CD28 or IL-2, IL-4 or IL-7 leads to activation and proliferation whereas other cytokines are ineffective (e.g. IFNγ, TNFα, IL-6, IL-10, IL-12). The triad of IL-2, IL-4 and IL-7 suggested involvement of the γ_c and cross-linking of γ_c by antibody was found to prevent the development of anergy to either soluble antigen or alloantigen.[92] Development of anergy to alloantigen was not prevented in the presence of MoAbs cross-linking IL-2Rα, IL-2Rβ, IL-4R or IL-7R.

A small number of studies have investigated whether CD25 MoAbs could lead to anergy by producing a relatively IL-2-deficient state or by producing tolerance through deletion of antigen specific cells. Prolonged graft survival of neural tissue implanted in rat brain could be achieved by a short course of CD25 MoAb therapy and subsequently tolerance to donor specific neural tissue implanted peripherally was demonstrated.[79] This rat model is a relatively weak alloantigenic stimulus because neural tissue does not normally express MHC antigens and the graft was implanted into a privileged site. In this model, an IL-2-blocking MoAb was necessary but without requiring depletion of IL-2Rα⁺ cells. The same tolerance could not be achieved by a short course of CsA. A more conventional induction of tolerance was achieved towards a fully allogeneic rat heart allograft by 10 days treatment with the CD25 MoAb (NDS 61) alone. This induced indefinite graft survival in 67% of rats, while the remainder rejected between 12-27 days compared to an untreated control survival of 7-11 days.[71] However a formal proof of tolerance by cell transfer studies or re-transplantation was not done.

In an autoimmune diabetic rat model, tolerance could be induced by using low doses of CsA together with a CD25 MoAb (ART-18). In syngeneic transplants within BB diabetic rats normoglycaemia was maintained for less than 20 days whereas treatment with subtherapeutic doses of CsA and ART-18 (1 mg/kg) maintained normoglycaemia for over 120 days. Rats showed evidence of tolerance in that they could be retransplanted with the same BB derived islet cell grafts without rejecting them, rejected third party islets grafts and transfer of splenocytes from tolerant to naive BB rats led to acceptance of syngeneic islet grafts in 75% of animals.[93]

Only CD25 MoAbs have been used in animal models of tolerance induction and it is obvious from the biology of the IL-2/IL-2R system that this leaves many pathways by which the blockade can be bypassed. To date, no animal transplantation studies have been reported on the use of CD122 MoAbs (anti-IL-2Rβ) alone or combined with CD25. It is interesting once again that different CD25 MoAbs with apparently the same properties have markedly different potencies. Thus ART-18 requires CsA at least in subtherapeutic doses for extended effect and cannot induce tolerance towards an allograft while NDS 61 is capable of doing so without requiring CsA.

HUMAN CLINICAL STUDIES USING CD25 MoABS

Quite large numbers of patients have now been treated with CD25 MoAbs in Phase I, II and III studies. The effect of CD25 MoAbs has been tested in transplantation with background immunosuppression of CsA, azathioprine (AZA) and prednisolone (P) or triple therapy and the CD25 MoAbs have either been added to this regime to make a quadruple therapy or used sequentially with the CD25 MoAb replacing CsA at the start of transplantation and introducing CsA when the MoAb therapy was finishing. Summaries of the clinical trials have been tabulated to allow comparison of the important issues and they will be dealt with organ by organ. CD25 MoAbs will be referred to by their original clone name and reference to their commercial name will be made where appropriate. All incidences of acute rejection (AR) and rejection rate (RR) per patient are reported for the first three months of transplantation.

RENAL TRANSPLANTATION

Despite the theoretical reasons against a CD25 MoAb reversing AR episodes, it has been tried as a therapy for rejections in renal transplant patients. 20 mg of 33B3-1 were given on the first two days followed by 10 mg daily for 8 days to 7 patients undergoing their first and 3 undergoing their second rejection. Rapid reversal occurred in 2 patients while creatinine levels stabilized in 4 patients and worsened in the remaining 4 patients. These results were regarded as relatively ineffective compared to conventional therapies for AR and were not pursued further.[94] Recently 14 patients with steroid resistant rejection episodes received B-B10 as a continuous infusion of 10 mg for 10 days and the rejections stabilized in 13 and remained stable for a year in 12/14. Biopsy proven resolution of rejection was obtained in 13 patients.[95] These recent results were surprising and further investigation in the treatment of AR by this particular CD25 MoAb seems warranted. No adverse events were reported with the use of either of these CD25

MoAbs during rejection episodes and no cytokine release syndrome occurred.

The use of CD25 MoAbs as prophylaxis in renal transplantation is shown in Table 3.6. The rat CD25 MoAb (33B3-1) was used first in renal transplantation and early studies established that a daily dose of 5 mg was insufficient but at 10 mg daily for 14 days there was a reduction of AR to about 30% in first renal transplant recipients. 33B3-1 was then tested in a randomized trial against anti-thymocyte globulin (ATG) and the incidence of AR once again was around 30% with no significant difference in AR compared to ATG.[96] More recently, another rat CD25 MoAb (LO-Tact-1) has also proven equal to ATG in a randomized trial but the frequency of AR was closer to 50%.[97] It was reported that soluble IL-2Rα levels were significantly lower in LO-Tact-1-treated patients than in the ATG controls which may mean that soluble IL-2Rα was removed from the circulation complexed to LO-Tact-1 or that the MoAb interfered with the assay.

Two randomized studies have compared CD25 MoAbs against triple therapy without any serotherapy. In the first, anti-Tac was used at half the CsA dosage of the control group (8mg/kg/day) during serotherapy. A pilot study using anti-Tac without any CsA saw an incidence of early rejection in 4 out of 5 patients and it was concluded that anti-Tac could not be used without CsA. Used together with CsA there was a 35% incidence of AR similar to previous CD25 MoAb studies and at a lower frequency than in controls but without achieving statistical significance. In the second, more recent study, a very low level of rejection was observed in both the CD25 MoAb (B-B10) and control groups in a trial with relatively small numbers of patients. 33B3-1 has proven to be slightly inferior to ATG when used in second kidney grafts or in combined kidney and pancreas grafts with ARs occurring nearly twice as frequently as in first grafts.[98,99] Despite the improvement in rejection frequencies and rate (Table 3.6) this has not yet translated into an improvement in one year graft survival.

All of these studies were free of any significant side effects associated with infusion of the CD25 MoAbs and better than the moderate side effects experienced by patients receiving ATG.[96] Infectious complications were not increased by the use of CD25 MoAbs compared to controls but on the other hand infectious complications were no less frequent than those seen with ATG,

Table 3.6. CD25 MoAb prophylaxis in human renal transplantation

Antibody	Dose mg	Days	Patient No.	% AR	RR	1 yr GS	Graft	HAMA %	Ref
B-B10 [A]	10	10	27	11.1		84	1st	60	[149]
Control			29	27.6		87			
33B3-1 [B]	5	14	9	44.4			1st	85	[102,103]
	10	14	48	27.1					
33B3-1 [B]	10	14	49	30.6	0.3	85	1st	81	[96]
ATG			46	26.1	0.3	85			
chRFT5 [C]	2.5-25	x 6	24	33.3	0.6	92	1st	0	[101]
chRFT2	5-30	x 6	15	64.0	1.4	87		0	
anti-Tac [D]	20	10	40	35.0	0.6	72	1st	70	[100]
Control	0		40	60.0	1.1	80			
LO-Tact-1 [E]	10	14	35	48.6	0.7	94	1st	89	[97,150]
ATG			40	40.0	0.5	90			
33B3-1 [F]	10	10	20	50.0			1st+Pan	65	[98]
ATG			20	30.0					
33B3-1 [G]	10	10	20	60.0	0.7	89	2nd	70	[99]
ATG			20	45.0	0.5	85			

Abbreviations: AR acute rejection, RR rejection rate per patient, GS graft survival, Pan pancreas.
[A] Dual therapy (CsA + P)
[B] Sequential triple therapy with CsA introduced on the day that serotherapy was stopped.
[C] Chimeric form of RFT5γ2a (SDZ CHI 621) given as infusions on days 0, 2, 6, 11, 17 and 24 post transplantation either with triple or dual therapy.
[D] 4/5 patients treated with anti-Tac without CsA experienced rapid AR. Triple therapy was used in the trial. CsA was at 4mg/kg/day during anti-Tac therapy and controls received 8mg/kg/day.
[E] Sequential triple therapy with introduction of AZA on day 45.
[F] Essentially triple therapy with CsA introduced as soon as creatinine level stabilised.
[G] As in [F] for combined kidney and pancreas graft.

even though the infections were thought to be less severe.[96] These findings suggest that the baseline immunosuppressive therapy is the most important determinant of infection while the contribution of 10-14 days of CD25 MoAb therapy has little impact on the overall susceptibility to infection.

The rapid development of human anti-monoclonal antibody (HAMA) responses could explain why a proportion of patients continue to experience rejection episodes despite treatment with CD25 MoAbs. Certainly HAMA responses occurred in the vast majority of patients (Table 3.6) and MoAb activity was neutralised in the presence of HAMA. HAMA was detectable during treatment in 40-65%, 40% and 44% of patients treated with 33B3-1, anti-Tac and LO-Tact-1, respectively. When anti-idiotype responses were measured they were found in 97% of 33B3-1[96] and 86% of anti-Tac patients.[100] HAMA responses could persist for up to six months but without interfering with the use of OKT3 for AR episodes. Some patients were able to be re-treated with 33B3-1 during re-grafting two to six months after its initial use.[98]

Chimerisation or humanization has been perceived to be the answer to HAMA responses and the curtailed action of murine MoAbs. A chimeric CD25 MoAb, chRFT5, has been submitted to Phase I studies in renal transplantation and has fulfilled the expectations of chimerisation.[101] It can be seen in Figure 3.2 that six doses of 5 mg of chRFT5 produced suppression of IL-2Rα+ cells for over a month with minimal effect on T cells generally. This favorably contrasts with the effect of OKT3 treatment where at 5 mg daily for 14 days there was severe depletion of all T cells including IL-2Rα+ T cells for 10 days followed by the rapid and exuberant reappearance of both T cells and IL-2Rα+ T cells even before OKT3 therapy had ceased. Therapy with murine CD25 MoAbs at doses of 10-20 mg are needed to achieve effective therapy that only lasts for 10-14 days. With chRFT5, the half-life in renal transplant patients was found to be 13 days, which is close to the half-life of IgG1 (21 days) and much greater than murine IgG MoAbs (24 hours) or the rat MoAb 33B3-1 (12 hours).[102] A difference in function of the chRFT5 compared to the murine anti-Tac was the complete suppression of IL-2Rα+. Throughout treatment with anti-Tac IL-2Rα+, cells could be detected at relatively high levels (15% compared to 22% in controls) despite the presence of anti-Tac in the serum[100] without being coated with mouse immunoglobulin. With chRFT5 the opposite was found in that IL-2Rα⁺ T cells were reduced in number and the remaining cells were coated with the chRFT5. The persistence of IL-2Rα⁺ T cells in anti-Tac-treated patients could be due to anti-Tac complexing preferentially with soluble IL-2R than to membrane IL-2R.

Despite the superior pharmacokinetic properties of chRFT5 there was an AR in 30% of patients similar to the frequency found using murine MoAbs (Table 3.6). These rejections occurred dur-

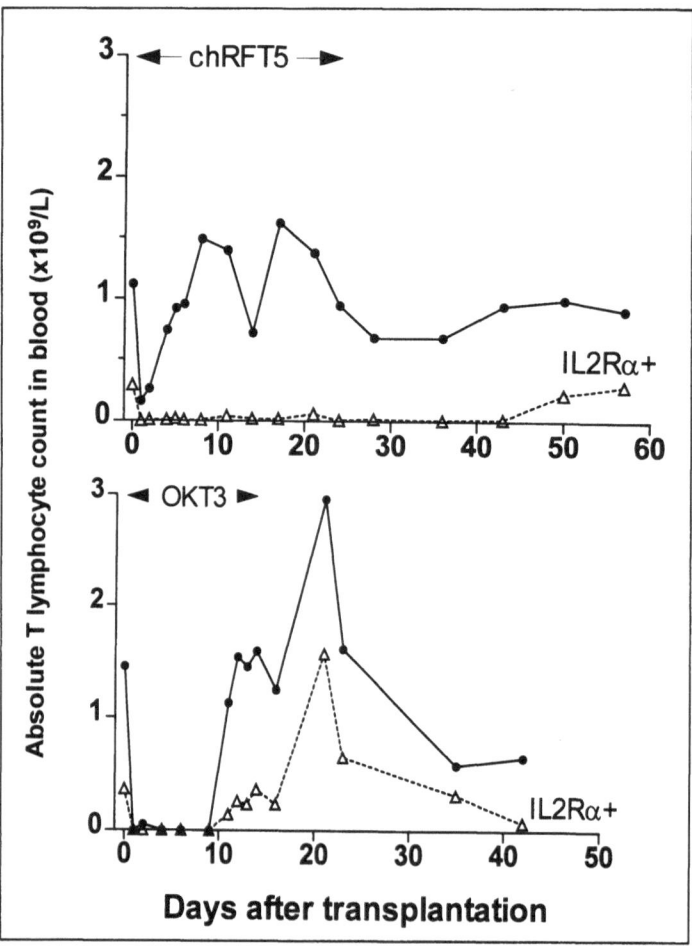

Fig. 3.2. Effects of chRFT5 and OKT3 on blood T cells. Solid circles and lines: T cells. Open triangles and dotted line: IL-2Rα⁺ T cells. ChRFT5 was given as six doses of 5 mg on days 0, 2, 6, 11, 17 and 24 of transplantation and OKT3 was given as 5 mg daily for 14 days from day 0 (pre-transplant).

ing the time that chRFT5 was present and functional in vivo[101] which suggested a bypassing of CD25 mediated blockade. It was possible though that the frequency of AR in the chimeric study was spurious because significantly more rejections occurred in patients with delayed primary function (6/8) than immediate primary function (2/16).[101] In delayed primary function protocol biopsies were performed and anti-rejection treatment given on the basis of weekly protocol biopsies. A cellular infiltrate suggesting rejection was the sole criterion upon which a decision to institute anti-rejection therapy was taken. Increased mononuclear cell infiltration, consistent with mild rejection, but in the absence of clinical evidence of rejection has been observed in renal and liver transplants.[103]

The remarkably long periods of IL-2Rα suppression with chRFT5 (up to 120 days) were not associated with any detectable HAMA or anti-idiotype responses and no increase in infectious complications. A worrying development was the appearance of two cases of EBV driven post-transplantation lymphoproliferative disease (PTLD). The PTLD arose 9 months post-transplant, were associated with prolonged IL-2Rα suppression and a delayed and prolonged lymphopoenia occurring only in patients treated by triple therapy but not dual therapy. This suggested an adverse interaction between chRFT5 and AZA or a global over-immunosuppression through the combination of four separate agents. PTLD has been reported in 1/106 patients treated with 33B3-1[102] which is a normal frequency for renal transplantation and another case of primary EBV infection was reported from 27 patients treated with B-B10.[104] The PTLD reported with B-B10 occurred 6 months post-transplantation. This unexpectedly high incidence of PTLD warns of the dangers associated with prolonged immunosuppression by CD25 MoAbs and care will be needed to monitor interactions with other immunosuppressive drugs.

LIVER TRANSPLANTATION

CD25 MoAbs have been used as part of quadruple therapy in liver transplantation and despite this intensive therapy the benefit of CD25 MoAbs has been equivocal. The first randomized study was performed using the rat MoAb, YTH 906 or Campath 6, against a control arm of triple therapy alone and it showed no benefit for the combination with YTH 906 in terms of rejection episodes, graft and patient survival or severity of histological rejection. A separate randomized trial using the rat MoAb LO-Tact-1 also failed to find any improvement in AR episodes compared to controls treated with triple therapy alone. However there was a trend in this study towards a better patient and graft survival at one year with fewer steroid resistant rejections and less severe rejection in the LO-Tact-1 treated group. A large number of patients were excluded from analysis in this study, particularly from the control group, because of early, non-immunological graft loss. One of the arms in this study was a group treated prophylactically with OKT3 and the results using OKT3 were similar to LO-Tact-1 but with a high incidence of CMV disease associated with OKT3 treatment. Although there was no diminution in rejection rates the authors raised the possibility that the histological evidence of graft infiltration by mononuclear cells may have influenced the diagnosis of rejection unduly in the case of LO-Tact-1 therapy.[105] This refers to the evidence seen in animal and human renal studies of graft infiltration not associated with clinical evidence of rejection.

Table 3.7. CD25 MoAb prophylaxis in human liver transplantation

Antibody	Dose mg	Days	No.	% AR	% 1 yr survival:		HAMA %	Ref
					Graft	Patient		
B-B10 [A]	10	12	33	12	91	91		107
ATG			33	24	94	94		
B-B10	Var	20	19	37				106
YTH906	25	10	49	61	74 [B]	78 [B]	43	152
			49	73	75 [B]	79 [B]		
LO-Tact-1	20	10	35	91	97	100	100	105
OKT3	5	10	37	81	86	86		
Control			29	96	75	79		

Baseline immunosuppression with triple therapy (CsA + AZA + Pred) and no sequential introduction of CsA or AZA.
[A] B-B10 given as a continuous infusion.
[B] To 6 months, not 1 year.

In a randomized trial there were fewer AR with B-B10 than ATG (Table 3.7). With B-B10 there was a lower post-operative temperature, higher bile production and faster fall in bilirubin than with ATG. Longer term outcome however did not differ between B-B10 and ATG with similarly good 1 year graft and patient survival and no difference in the incidence of infections. Cellular infiltration of the graft had been seen in 27% of protocol biopsies not associated with clinical evidence of rejection in a pilot study.[106] In the randomized study there was a similar high incidence of histological rejection in the B-B10 group and at a higher level 27/33 (82%) than seen with ATG 12/33 (36%). Soluble IL-2R rose after treatment with B-B10 and was detectable during therapy.[107]

HAMA responses to mouse immunoglobulin were frequent (Table 3.7) and with LO-Tact-1 developed on days 10, 15 and 20 in 31%, 61% and 100% of which 8, 15 and 69% contained anti-idiotypic antibodies respectively. Once again there was no problem using OKT3 after LO-Tact-1.

GRAFT VERSUS HOST DISEASE (GVHD)

In animal studies CD25 MoAbs had proved effective prophylactically in local GVHD or GVHD arising across minor histocompatibility barriers but not in reversing ongoing GVHD (Table 3.4). It was logical therefore to use CD25 MoAbs in GVHD arising in matched related donors (MRD) differing across minor MHC antigens but it was not expected that CD25 MoAb could successfully reverse ongoing GVHD.

TREATMENT OF ACUTE GVHD

Allogeneic bone marrow transplantation (BMT) performed without T-cell depletion of the BMT leads to $\geq$ Grade II GVHD in 20-30% of MRD and rising to 70-90% in partially matched related donors (PMRD) or matched unrelated donors (MUD) despite prophylaxis with CsA and methotrexate (MTX). Only half of the patients with GVHD will have durable responses to steroids, further CsA or ATG. Uncontrolled GVHD is the main cause of death in these patients. The effect of CD25 MoAbs was examined in patients with steroid resistant GVHD being treated mostly for leukemia. The results of these studies are shown in Table 3.8 and are dominated by the use of B-B10. B-B10 not only dominates numerically but also in superior results compared with the

Table 3.8. CD25 MoAb therapy of acute GVHD in BMT

Antibody	MoAb therapy: Dose [A]	Days	Outcome of therapy as %: No	CR [B]	Relapse [C]	Death	Ref
B-B10	0.2-0.4	12 - 70	15	80	46	33	109
B-B10	5	20 [D]	32	66	48	56	152
B-B10	10	20 [E]	31	55	35	71	153
B-B10	10	20 [D]	99	51	46	55	108
B-B10	5	20 [D]	14	28	25	71	110
HAT [F]	0.5-1.5	1	19	16	100	95	111
2A3	0.1-1.0	7	10	10	0	90	112

[A] Given as mg/day or in decimal range as mg/kg/day
[B] Complete remission
[C] Relapse includes chronic GVHD
[D] Given daily for 10 days then alternate days till day 20
[E] 10 mg daily for 3 days, then 5 mg daily for 7 days and then on alternate days to day 20
[F] Humanized anti-Tac

Table 3.9. MHC matching and GVHD grades in acute GVHD

Antibody	CR %	MHC matching (%): MRD	PMRD	MUD/PMUD	GVHD grades as %: II	III	IV	HAMA	Ref
B-B10	80	–	100	–	27	71	7	na	109
B-B10	66	72	16	12 / –	50	34	16	7	152
B-B10	55	97	–	3 / –				na	153
B-B10	51	70	11	19 / –	57	32	11	20	108
B-B10	28	50	–	36 / 14	7	29	64	na	110
HAT [A]	16	32	5	47 / 16	5	63	32	0	111
2A3	10	36	64	–	36	46	18	50	112

Abbreviations—MRD: matched related donor, PMRD: partly matched related donor, MUD/PMUD: matched and partly matched unrelated donor.
[A] One patient with Grade I GVHD who achieved a CR has been removed because no steroids were given.

other two CD25 MoAbs including the humanized anti-Tac (HAT). Better results were achieved in MRD than PMRD or MUD patients and this partly explains the superiority of B-B10 (Table 3.9). Response to treatment with B-B10 was more likely if treatment occurred within a month of the start of GVHD and was less likely with GVHD affecting the liver.[108] The decreased responsiveness of GVHD with delay in starting treatment by B-B10 may be due to a change in the nature of the immune response with time making it less dependent on IL-2 or simply that with time the patient's general condition deteriorates.

The best results were achieved in a group of children at high risk of GVHD receiving PMRD bone marrow for correction of congenital immunodeficiency disease.[109] The intention in this study was to treat steroid resistant GVHD early (mean of 8 days from start of GVHD) and intensively (mean duration of 26 days) with B-B10. Unlike previous studies, there was no evidence of organ resistance and complete responses (CR) were seen in 80% of skin, 94% of gut and 100% of liver GVHD. However liver disease was reported to be mild in all cases. Six patients who relapsed were returned to CR with a second course of B-B10 and one of two who relapsed for a second time responded to a third course of B-B10. No loss of efficacy was seen despite repeated treatments over 70 days.

The studies that were comparable in terms of severity of GVHD and proportions of MRD to PMRD or MUD using different types of CD25 MoAb still showed a superiority for B-B10 over HAT and 2A3.[110-112] Particularly disappointing was the low CR rate and poor survival of patients treated with HAT despite receiving treatment within a favorable time period from the start of GVHD (< 1 month) and, from the evidence of pharmacokinetic studies, for longer than was achievable by B-B10 in its murine form. Eight patients achieving any response to one infusion of HAT were retreated but none achieved a CR with a second infusion. Coating of IL-2Rα⁺ cells with HAT occurred without evidence of depletion.[111] Treatment of GVHD with 2A3 was ineffective but unusually for CD25 MoAbs it induced relatively frequent side effects during infusion (15%) consisting of hypertension, fever, respiratory distress, hypotension and chills[112] as well as a high frequency of HAMA responses (50%) for patients with GVHD.

PROPHYLAXIS OF GVHD

All of the prophylactic studies involved treatment of groups of
BMT patients at high risk of GVHD (PMRD and MUD) and
included one randomized trial while the remainder were compared
against historical controls (H-control). None of the CD25 MoAbs
were effective in reducing the frequency GVHD or mortality from
this complication even though they produced a slight delay in the
time to GVHD (Table 3.10). GVHD occurred in 10 patients even
while they were receiving LO-Tact-1 therapy.[113] Not only was the
prophylactic use of CD25 MoAbs ineffective but there was evidence of a detrimental effect similar to that seen with T cell depleted BMT. In a randomized trial, the incidence of leukemia relapse was higher in the CD25 MoAb treated group (33B3-1 = 42%;
controls = 20%) and disease free survival (DFS) was lower
(33B3-1 = 41%; control = 66.2%). Cox regression analysis showed
that the two factors influencing the relapse rate of the underlying
leukemia were 33B3-1 and chronic GVHD while DFS related to
33B3-1 and acute GVHD. These results support the hypothesis

Table 3.10. Prophylactic CD25 mab therapy in bone marrow
transplantation

Antibody	MoAb therapy:		No.	Occurrence and effects of GVHD:			Ref
	Dose [A]	Day		≥ 2 Grade %	Mean day	Mortality %	
33B3-1 [B]	20	0 - 2	51	38	36	28	114,154
	10	3 - 28					
Control			50	46	25	20	
B-B10	10	0 - 40	8	50		25	155
LO-Tact-1	0.2	7 - 28	15	40	13	27	113
	0.4	-1 - 28	12	67	31	8	
H-Control			30	27	19	7	
2A3	1.0	-1	10	70	20	80	115
	0.5	0-19					
H-Control			31	87	13	94	

All patients received CsA and methotrexate prophylaxis.
[A] Given as mg/day or in decimal range as mg/kg/day
[B] Chronic GVHD was the same in both groups.

that removal of cells capable of inducing acute or chronic GVHD also removes cells active in a graft-versus-leukemia effect.[114] Once again 2A3 was particularly immunogenic with HAMA occurring in 40% of patients.[115]

HEART TRANSPLANTATION

Only B-B10 has been used in heart transplants (Table 3.11). Although rejection episodes were significantly more frequent in the B-B10 treated group than with ATG, no grafts were lost and the infection rate was significantly lower with B-B10 (15% versus 54% respectively).[116] Monitoring of rejections in heart transplantation relies heavily on repeated endomyocardial biopsies and grading of the cellular infiltrate. Repeated finding of cellular infiltrates in CD25 MoAb-treated grafts in the absence of clinical rejection will have to be taken into consideration in evaluating efficacy in heart transplants.

Three heart transplant patients with repeated rejection episodes treated by pulsed steroids, OKT3 and ATG were treated for their 4th and 5th rejection episodes with B-B10 and improvement in histological rejection was reported after 12 days of treatment. No clinical information was given.[117]

WHAT MAKES A THERAPEUTICALLY EFFECTIVE CD25 MOAB?

Table 3.12 compares properties of the different CD25 MoAbs used in clinical studies. All of these MoAbs recognize the same CD25A, IL-2 binding epitope[118] and consequently this is not a discriminant of clinical efficacy although it implies that MoAbs recognizing epitopes CD25B and CD25C are ineffective. Clinical efficacy of CD25 MoAbs has been ranked from B-B10 (the most

---

Table 3.11. CD25 MoAb prophylaxis in human heart transplantation

Antibody	Dose mg	Days	No.	% AR	% Survival to 6 mo: Graft	Patient	Ref
B-B10	10	8	13	90	100	100	116
ATG			14	35	86	86	

Legend as for liver transplantation.

Table 3.12. Characteristics of CD25 MoAbs used in clinical trials

MoAbs	IgG subclass: Rodent [A]	Human Fc	Affinity Kd (nM)	Inhibition of: IC$_{50}$ (nM) [B]	MLR	IL-2 growth	ADCC	Ref
B-B10	IgG1	IgG1	2	0.04	++ [C]	++	–	156
33B3-1	IgG2a rat	–	0.3	?	+	++	?	22
RFT5γ2a	IgG2a	IgG1 [D]	0.1	0.03	+	+++	–	
anti-Tac	IgG2a	IgG1 [E]	1	0.2	+	++	–	125
LO-Tact-1	IgG2b rat	–	?	>100	+++	?	+	105
2A3	IgG1	–	0.7	3.0	+	++	–	115
YTH 906	IgG2b rat	–	?	?	+++	+	+	74

All mabs inhibit IL-2 binding to its receptor and all recognise the A epitope.
  However YTH 906 is only partially cross-blocking with RFT5γ2a which cross
  blocks completely with 33B3-1, B-B10 and anti-Tac.
[A] Mouse mabs unless otherwise indicated.
[B] 50% killing of a CD25 expressing cell line (L540) by ricin A chain conjugates.[157]
[C] Inhibits MLR when added on day 4.
[D] Chimerised RFT5γ2a. All chimeric/humanized moabs have ADCC activity.
[E] Humanized anti-Tac has an affinity of 3nM - a three fold loss during
  humanization.[125]

widely used and frequently effective MoAb) through to 2A3 and
YTH 906 (of no benefit clinically). On this basis, features that
may be relevant to therapeutic efficacy have been evaluated.

1. Function of the constant Fc portion of the rodent IgG does
not seem of primary importance because rat IgG2b and murine
IgG1 carry the most and least potent effector function yet this
does not correlate at all with clinical efficacy. Switching of the
murine constant region to human IgG1 by genetic engineering
should make murine MoAbs like B-B10 as effective as rat IgG2b.

2. Affinity of the MoAbs does not correlate with clinical
efficacy.

3. The ability of MoAbs to internalize the IL-2R was demonstrated sensitively by a cytotoxic assay using ricin conjugated antibodies. This assay may rank effective MoAbs with B-B10 being
potent in this assay and 2A3 relatively weak. The value obtained
for LO-Tact-1 may be misleading because the ricin conjugate was
attached to anti-mouse IgG which although cross-reacting with rat
IgG may not have functioned as effectively.

4. Inhibition of the mixed lymphocyte reaction (MLR) does not correlate with clinical efficacy. The ineffective MoAb, YTH 906, is a potent inhibitor of the MLR-like LO-Tact-1. The potency of these rat IgG2b MoAbs may be related to effective ADCC activity in vitro which is lacking in most of the murine MoAbs. B-B10 was selected because of its ability to inhibit when added late to an MLR but in this respect it does not differ from RFT5.

5. Inhibition of IL-2 driven proliferation is only partly related to clinical activity and although YTH 906 is weak at inhibiting IL-2 driven proliferation this is not so for 2A3.

The features above define what is necessary for a clinically effective MoAb but are not sufficient in themselves. It is likely that the fine specificity of the binding site on the IL-2Rα will be critical for clinical activity. All CD25 MoAbs have a single binding site curve and none show biphasic curves like IL-2. The ability to inhibit high affinity binding although important is not sufficient because 2A3 is capable of inhibiting IL-2 binding under high affinity binding conditions and yet is ineffective clinically.[119] Preferential binding to the membrane bound IL-2Rα rather than the released soluble IL-2Rα or binding that interferes with or disrupts the assembly of the high affinity IL-2αβγ could contribute to make one MoAb more effective than another.

GENETICALLY ENGINEERED MoABS

Several CD25 MoAbs have been chimerised (RFT5γ2a, AHT54, AHT107, 2C8, 3G10 and MAK179)[120-124] or humanized (anti-Tac and B-B10)[125,126] and all have used the human IgG1 heavy and κ light chains. Without exception, the human IgG1 heavy chain has endowed the chimeric or humanized MoAb with ADCC but not complement dependent cytotoxicity against a variety of targets expressing IL-2Rα. One MoAb, AHT107, which unlike the rest was unable to block IL-2 mediated proliferation gained this after chimerisation and was probably due to acquired ADCC activity since this did not occur in cell systems devoid of effector cells.[121] Two MoAbs recognizing the IL-2Rβ chain have been chimerised (A41)[127] and humanized (Mikβ1)[128] respectively and like the CD25 MoAbs they have used IgG1κ. The humanized Mikβ1 inhibits LGL activity mediated by IL-2 and in certain systems augments ADCC killing of IL-2Rβ expressing cells.[128] HAT and chRFT5 that have been used clinically are not immunogenic in a setting of GVHD and renal transplantation respectively and the latter may have evidence of effector function in vivo. Both HAT and chRFT5 have prolonged half lives of 4 and 13 days respectively.[101,111] All these features indicate that the goal of genetic engineering has been achieved. However, in the case of HAT this has not managed to make it a better MoAb clinically than B-B10 in treating GVHD. It is still too early to assess the value of chRFT5 but in the Phase I/II studies the extension of its half-life and prolonged activity has not improved on the results achieved with the rat MoAb 33B3-1. Overlong action of the chRFT5 may have led to interaction with other immunosuppressive agents and increased susceptibility to EBV-driven proliferation. A controlled randomized trial with suppression of the IL-2Rα+ T cells will determine the value of chimerisation in a MoAb that was selected for all the characteristics thought necessary for clinical effectiveness. Since half the CD8 cells express IL-2Rβγ chains (Table 3.3), blockade of CD25 will not inhibit their expansion and these cells may form part of the graft infiltrate seen with CD25 MoAb therapy and lead to the slightly delayed graft rejection seen with both rodent and chimeric CD25 MoAbs. In this scenario class I MHC mismatches would be of more significance than class II.

FUTURE DEVELOPMENTS

From our understanding of the biology of the IL-2/IL-2R system it is evident that the use of CD25 MoAbs alone are not going to be able to block IL-2-driven clonal expansion and have not been able to delete all IL-2Rα+ cells in the clinic. Targeting the high affinity IL-2Rαβγ complex should be more effective. Attempts at such targeting were made using IL-2 in the form of an immunotoxin consisting of IL-2 linked directly to diphtheria toxin (DT) in a fusion protein (IL-2DT). IL-2DT internalizes like IL-2 and the DT kills the cell leading to elimination of T cells expressing IL-2Rαβγ. Delayed type hypersensitivity was suppressed by IL-2DT in mice even in the presence of relatively high titres of antibody to diphtheria toxoid[129] and it prolonged cardiac graft survival in mice, in some cases indefinitely. For mice there was a large therapeutic margin with toxicity requiring much higher doses than for therapeutic effect. Toxicity was primarily renal. Mice did not develop neutralizing antibodies until well after the therapeutic effect had been achieved.[130] The problem with this approach when extended to man has been the much greater toxicity of IL-2DT similar to most types of immunotoxin. The main problem with IL-2DT was due to allergic reactions in humans but it could also cause a vascular leak syndrome.[131] In an attempt to avoid the side effects associated with toxins, a human IgM was genetically constructed so that the antigen binding sites (Fv) of the antibody were replaced by IL-2. This combination of high affinity binding by IL-2 with IgM mediated complement fixation was designed to cause lysis of activated cells[132] but the physical combination of the relatively insoluble IgM with ten hydrophobic IL-2 molecules created a construct that was poorly soluble in aqueous solutions.

Possibilities of using MoAbs to the other IL-2R chains are being explored. The γ_c chain is an inappropriate target on its own because it does not bind IL-2 directly and it is so widely expressed that the specificity associated with IL-2Rα targeting would be lost. Indeed effective targeting of the γ_c could be devastatingly immunosuppressive since rendering this chain non-functional could lead to an X-SCID like syndrome. CD122 MoAbs recognizing the IL-2Rβ chain are available[133-135] but have not been used in transplant studies largely through a lack of inhibitory activity on their own. Like CD25 MoAbs, there are several epitopes recognized by CD122 MoAbs only some of which affect IL-2 binding. Inhibition of IL-2-driven proliferation by CD25 MoAbs is potentiated by the simultaneous presence of CD122 MoAbs but this interaction is decreased in the presence of high amounts of IL-2Rα[135] which may be due to stoichometric interference since HAT inhibits CD122 (Mikβ1) binding to PHA blasts when there is an excess of IL-2Rα chain expression.[128] The combined blockade by CD25 and CD122 MoAbs starts to affect cells not involved in solid organ transplant rejection such as NK cells and consequently broadens the immunosuppression. For example, a CD122 MoAb TU27 could not inhibit the induction of CTL alone but could in combination with a CD25 MoAb and the combination inhibited expansion of CD4 and CD8[hi] cells in an MLR with greater resistance to the addition of exogenous IL-2 but the combination also led to a decrease in NK cells not seen with CD25 MoAbs alone.[65] Nonetheless this cooperation between CD25 and CD122 MoAbs might start to rationalize the effectiveness of anti-IL-2R MoAbs thus avoiding the arbitrary superiority of one CD25 MoAb over another due to fine specificity of its binding to the IL-2Rα chain. Construction of bispecific MoAbs (bi-MoAbs) is a method which might allow selectivity for the high affinity IL-2Rαβγ complex and minimize interaction with the IL-2Rβγ complex expressed on CD8 cells and NK cells. Bi-MoAbs constructed from Fab′ fragments of CD25 (33B3-1) and CD122 (A41) MoAbs have approached the functionality of IL-2 with both low and high affinity binding to T cells. High affinity binding does not occur on cells kept at 4°C but does at 37°C suggesting that dynamic association of the IL-2R chains is required. Bi-MoAbs were 5- to 10-fold more potent than the combined presence of the individual CD25 and CD122 MoAbs.[136] Similar use of bi-MoAbs to target IL-2Rβγ chains would be counter productive and lead to incessant proliferation since cross-linking these molecules is essentially the function of IL-2.

The unraveling of the IL-2/IL-2R system has made a fascinating and changing story ever since its discovery. As more reagents become available to interfere with its function we are acquiring very potent immunosuppressive agents and great care will have to be taken in their application and how they are used in combination with conventional immunosuppressive drugs. In the immediate future, effective CD25 MoAbs will further reduce AR episodes in many solid organ transplants and provide an effective means of reversing GVHD used initially alone or with steroids. In the more distant future, combination of CD25 and CD122 MoAbs may provide an effective induction to transplantation with sequential introduction of other immunosuppressive drugs as serotherapy is phased out. It will be intriguing to see whether combinations of CD25 and CD122 MoAbs may more effectively achieve tolerance than CD25 MoAbs alone.

REFERENCES

1. Morgan DA, Ruscetti FW and Gallo RC. Selective in vitro growth of T-lymphocytes from normal human bone marrow. Science 1976; 193:1007-1008.
2. Leonard WJ, Depper JM, Uchiyama T, Smith KA, Waldmann TA and Greene WC. A monoclonal antibody that appears to recognize the receptor for human T-cell growth factor; partial characterization of the receptor. Nature 1982; 300:267-269.
3. Jenkinson EJ, Kingston R and Owen JJ. Importance of IL-2 receptors in intrathymic generation of cells expressing T-cell receptors. Nature 1987; 329:160-162.

4. Tanaka T, Takeuchi Y, Shiohara T et al. In utero treatment with monoclonal antibody to IL-2 receptor beta-chain completely abrogates development of Thy-1+ dendritic epidermal cells. Int Immunol 1992; 4:487-491.

5. Hefeneider S, Conlon P, Henney C and Gillis S. In vivo interleukin 2 administration augments the generation of alloreactive cytolytic T lymphocytes and resident natural killer cells. J Immunol 1983; 130:222-227.

6. Handa K, Suzuki R, Matsui H, Shimizu Y and Kumagai K. Natural killer (NK) cells as a responder to interleukin-2 (rIL-2). II. rIL-2-induce interferon gamma production. J Immunol 1983; 130:988-992.

7. Mule JJ, Shu S and Rosenberg SA. The anti-tumour efficacy of lymphokine-activated killer cells and recombinant interleukin 2 in vivo. J Immunol 1984; 135:646-652.

8. Rosenstein M, Yron I, Kaufmann Y and Rosenberg SA. Lymphokine activated killer cells: lysis of fresh syngeneic NK-resistant murine tumor cells by lymphocytes cultured in interleukin-2. Cancer Res 1984; 44:1946-1953.

9. Burdach S, Shatsky M, Wagenhorst B and Levitt L. Receptor specific modulation of myelopoiesis by recombinant DNA-derived IL-2. J Immunol 1987; 139:452-458.

10. Uchiyama T, Nelson DL, Fleisher TA and Waldmann TA. A monoclonal antibody (anti-Tac) reactive with activated and functionally mature human T cells. II. Expression of Tac antigen on activated cytotoxic killer T cells, suppressor cells, and on one of two types of helper T cells. J Immunol 1981; 126:1398-1403.

11. Hatakeyama M, Tsudo M, Minamoto S et al. Interleukin-2 receptor β chain gene: Generation of three receptor forms by cloned human α and β chain cDNA's. Science 1989;244:551-556.

12. Tsudo M, Karasuyama H, Kitamura F, Nagakaka Y, Tanaka T and Miyasaka M. The IL-2 receptor β chain (p70): Ligand binding ability of the cDNA-encoding membrane and secreted forms. J Immunol 1990; 145:599-606.

13. Minamoto S, Mori H, Hatakeyama M et al. Characterisation of the heterodimeric complex of human IL-2 receptor αβ chains reconstituted in a mouse fibroblast cell line, L929. J Immunol 1990; 145:2177-2182.

14. Voss SD, Robb RJ, Weil-Hillman G et al. Increased expression of the interleukin 2 (IL-2) receptor β chain (p70) on CD56$^+$ natural killer cells after in vivo IL-2 therapy: p70 expression does not alone predict the level of intermediate affinity IL-2 binding. J Exp Med 1990; 172:1101-1114.

15. Takeshita T, Ohtani K, Asao H, Kumaki S, Nakamura M and Sugamura K. An associated molecule, p64, with IL-2 receptor β chain. J Immunol 1992; 148:2154-2158.

16. Takeshita T, Asao H, Suzuki J and Sugamura K. An associated molecule, p64, with high affinity IL-2 receptor. Int Immunol 1990; 2:477-480.
17. Taniguchi T, Matsui H, Fujita T et al. Structure and expression of a cloned cDNA for human interleukin-2. Nature 1983; 302:305-310.
18. Nakamura Y, Russell SM, Mess SA et al. Heterodimerization of the IL-2 receptor beta- and gamma-chain cytoplasmic domains is required for signaling. Nature 1994; 369:330-333.
19. Nelson BH, Lord JD and Greenberg PD. Cytoplasmic domains of the interleukin-2 receptor beta and gamma chains mediate the signal for T-cell proliferation. Nature 1994; 369:333-336.
20. Rubin LA, Jay G and Nelson DL. The released interleukin-2 receptor binds interleukin-2 efficiently. J Immunol 1986; 137:3841-3844.
21. Siegel JP, Sharon M, Smith PL and Leonard WJ. The IL-2 receptor β chain (p70):role in mediating signals for LAK, NK and proliferative activities. Science 1987; 238:75-78.
22. Audrain M, Boeffard F, Soulillou JP and Jacques Y. Synergistic action of monoclonal antibodies directed at p55 and p75 chains of the human IL-2-receptor. J Immunol 1991; 146:884-892.
23. Bamford RN, Grant AJ, Burton JD et al. The interleukin (IL) 2 receptor beta chain is shared by IL-2 and a cytokine, provisionally designated IL-T, that stimulates T-cell proliferation and the induction of lymphokine-activated killer cells. Proc Natl Acad Sci USA 1994; 91:4940-4944.
24. Giri JG, Ahdieh M, Eisenman J et al. Utilization of the beta and gamma chains of the IL-2 receptor by the novel cytokine IL-15. EMBO J 1994; 13:2822-2830.
25. Grabstein KH, Eisenman J, Shanebeck K et al. Cloning of a T cell growth factor that interacts with the β chain of the interleukin-2 receptor. Science 1994; 264:965-968.
26. Takeshita T, Asao H, Ohtani K et al. Cloning of the gamma chain of the human IL-2 receptor. Science 1992; 257:379-382.
27. Kondo M, Takeshita T, Ishii N et al. Sharing of the interleukin-2 (IL-2) receptor gamma chain between receptors for IL-2 and IL-4 [see comments]. Science 1993; 262:1874-1877.
28. Russell SM, Keegan AD, Harada N et al. Interleukin-2 receptor gamma chain: a functional component of the interleukin-4 receptor [see comments]. Science 1993; 262:1880-1883.
29. Noguchi M, Nakamura Y, Russell SM et al. Interleukin-2 receptor γ chain: a functional component of the interleukin-7 receptor. Science 1993; 262:1877-1880.
30. Kondo M, Takeshita T, Higuchi M et al. Functional participation of the IL-2 receptor gamma chain in IL-7 receptor complexes. Science 1994; 263:1453-1454.

31. Fernandez-Botran R, Sanders VM and Vitetta ES. Interactions between receptors for interleukin 2 and interleukin 4 on lines of helper T cells (HT-2) and B lymphoma cells (BCL1). J Exp Med 1989; 169:379-391.
32. Martinez OM, Gibbons RS, Garovoy MR and Aronson FR. IL-4 inhibits IL-2 receptor expression and IL-2-dependent proliferation of human T cells. J Immunol 1990; 144:2211-2215.
33. Lee HK, Xia X and Choi YS. IL-4 blocks the up-regulation of IL-2 receptors induced by IL-2 in normal human B cells. J Immunol 1990; 144:3431-3436.
34. Defrance T, Vanbervliet B, Aubry JP and Banchereau J. Interleukin 4 inhibits the proliferation but not the differentiation of activated human B cells in response to interleukin 2. J Exp Med 1988; 168:1321-1337.
35. Vazquez A, Mills S and Maizel A. Modulation of IL-2-induced human B cell proliferation in the presence of human 50-kDa B cell growth factor and IL-4. J Immunol 1989; 142:94-99.
36. Migliorati G, Cardinali L and Riccardi C. Effect of interleukin-4 on interleukin-2-dependent generation of natural killer cells. Cell Immunol 1991; 136:194-207.
37. Muegge K, Vila MP and Durum SK. Interleukin-7:A cofactor for V(D)J rearrangement of the T cell receptor β chain. Science 1993; 261:93-95.
38. Watson JD, Morrissey PJ, Namen AE, Conlon PJ and Widmer MB. Effect of IL-7 on the growth of fetal thymocytes in culture. J Immunol 1989; 143:1215-1222.
39. Murray R, Suda T, Wrighton N, Lee F and Zlotnik A. IL-7 is a growth and maintenance factor for mature and immature thymocyte subsets. Int Immunol 1989; 1:526-531.
40. Uckun FM. Interleukin 7 receptor engagement stimulates tyrosine phosphorylation, inositol phospholipid turnover, proliferation, and selective differentiation to the CD4 lineage by human fetal thymocytes. Proc Natl Acad Sci USA 1991; 88:6323-6327.
41. Chazen GD. Interleukin 7 is a T-cell growth factor. Proc Natl Acad Sci USA 1989; 86:5923-5927.
42. Londei M, Verhoef A, Hawrylowicz C, Groves J, DeBerardinis P and Feldmann M. Interleukin 7 is a growth factor for mature human T cells. Eur J Immunol 1990; 20:425-428.
43. Morrissey PJ. Recombinant interleukin 7, pre-B cell growth factor, has costimulatory activity on purified mature T cells. J Exp Med 1989; 169:707-716.
44. Carding SR, Hayday AC and Bottomly K. Cytokines in T-cell development. Immunol Today 1991; 12:239-245.
45. Foxwell BM, Willcocks JL, Taylor-Fishwick DA, Kulig K, Ryffel B and Londei M. Inhibition of activation-induced changes in the structure of the T cell interleukin-7 receptor by cyclosporin A and

FK506. Eur J Immunol 1993; 23:85-89.

46. Noguchi M, Yi H, Rosenblatt HM et al. Interleukin-2 receptor ψ chain mutation results in X-linked severe combined immunodeficiency in humans. Cell 1993; 73:147-157.

47. Saltzman EM, Thom RR and Casnellie JE. Activation of a tyrosine protein kinase is an early event in the stimulation of T lymphocytes by interleukin-2. J Biol Chem 1988; 263:6956-6959.

48. Cantrell DA and Smith KA. The interleukin-2 T-cell system:a new cell growth model. Science 1984; 224:1312-1316.

49. Minami Y, Kono T, Miyazaki T and Taniguchi T. The IL-2 receptor complex:its structure, function, and target genes. [Review]. Ann Rev Immunol 1993; 11:245-268.

50. Roussel MF, Cleveland JL, Shurtleff SA and Sherr CJ. Myc rescue of a mutant CSF-1 receptor impaired in mitogenic signaling. Nature 1991; 353:361-363.

51. Schorle H, Holtschke T, Hunig T, Schimpl A and Horak I. Development and function of T cells in mice rendered interleukin-2 deficient by gene targeting. Nature 1991; 352:621-624.

52. Kuhn R, Rajewsky K and Muller W. Generation and analysis of interleukin-4 deficient mice. Science 1991; 254:707-710.

53. Kopf M, Le Gros G, Bachmann M, Lamers MC, Bluethmann H and Kohler G. Disruption of the murine IL-4 gene blocks the Th2 cytokine responses. Nature 1993; 362:245-247.

54. Sadlack B, Merz H, Schorle H, Schimpl A, Feller AC and Horak I. Ulcerative colitis-like disease in mice with a disrupted interleukin-2 gene. Cell 1993; 75:253-261.

55. DiSanto JP, Keever CA, Small TN, Nichols GL, O'Reilly RJ and Flomenberg N. Absence of interleukin 2 production in a severe combined immunodeficiency disease syndrome with T cells. J Exp Med 1990; 171:1697-1704.

56. Katsuki M, Kimura M, Ohta M et al. Lymphocyte infiltration into cerebellum in transgenic mice carrying human IL-2 gene. Int Immunol 1989; 1:214-218.

57. Ishida Y, Nishi M, Taguchi O et al. Effects of the deregulated expression of human interleukin-2 in transgenic mice. Int Immunol 1989; 1:113-120.

58. Boulay JL and Paul WE. The interleukin-4-related lymphokines and their binding to hematopoietin receptors. J Biol Chem 1992; 267:20525-20528.

59. Bazan JF. Structural design and molecular evolution of a cytokine receptor superfamily. Proc Natl Acad Sci USA 1990; 87:6934-6938.

60. Kanakura Y, Sugahara H, Mitsui H et al. Functional expression of interleukin 2 receptor in a human factor-dependent megakaryoblastic leukemia cell line:Evidence that granulocyte-macrophage colony-stimulating factor inhibits interleukin 2 binding to its receptor. Cancer Res 1993; 53:675-680.

61. Cao X, Kozak CA, Liu YJ, Noguchi M, O'Connell E and Leonard WJ. Characterization of cDNAs encoding the murine interleukin 2 receptor (IL-2R) gamma chain: chromosomal mapping and tissue specificity of IL-2R gamma chain expression. Proc Natl Acad Sci USA 1993; 90:8464-8468.

62. Sudo T. Expression and function of the interleukin 7 receptor in murine lymphocytes. Proc Natl Acad Sci USA 1993; 90:9125-9129.

63. Grabstein KH, Waldschmidt TJ, Finkelman FD et al. Inhibition of murine B and T lymphopoiesis in vivo by an anti-interleukin 7 monoclonal antibody. J Exp Med 1993; 178:257-264.

64. Amlot PL, Rawlings E, Tahami F and Chinn D. Concordant and discordant expression of activation antigens on human T cells (TCRab) from umbilical cord, adult blood and lymphoid tissue measured by two colour flow cytometry. Clin Exp Immunol 1995; (in press)

65. Niguma T, Sakagami K, Kawamura T et al. Expression of the interleukin 2 receptor beta chain (p75) in renal transplantation—applicability of anti-interleukin-2 receptor beta chain monoclonal antibody. Transplantation 1991; 52:296-302.

66. Ishii N, Takeshita T, Kimura Y et al. Expression of the IL-2 receptor γ chain on various populations in human peripheral blood. Int Immunol 1994; 6:1273-1277.

67. Plaisance S, Rubinstein E, Alileche A et al. Expression of the interleukin-2 receptor on human fibroblasts and its biological significance. Int Immunol 1992; 4:739-746.

68. Caux C, Massacrier C, Vanbervliet B et al. Activation of human dendritic cells through CD40 cross-linking. J Exp Med 1994; 180:1263.

69. Kupiec-Weglinski JW, Diamantstein T and Tilney NL. Interleukin 2 receptor-targeted therapy–rationale and applications in organ transplantation. Transplantation 1988; 46:785-792.

70. Tellides G, Dallman MJ and Morris PJ. Synergistic interaction of cyclosporine A with interleukin 2 receptor monoclonal antibody therapy. Transplant Proc 1988; 20:202-208.

71. Tellides G, Dallman MJ and Morris PJ. NDS 61, a new monoclonal antibody to the rat interleukin 2 receptor (IL-2R) induces long term allograft survival. British Journal of Surgery 1987; 74:1145-1146.

72. Reed MH, Shapiro ME, Strom TB et al. Prolongation of primate renal allograft survival by anti-Tac, an anti-human IL-2 receptor monoclonal antibody. Transplantation 1989; 47:55-59.

73. Brown PS, Jr., Parenteau GL, Dirbas FM et al. Anti-Tac-H, a humanized antibody to the interleukin 2 receptor, prolongs primate cardiac allograft survival. Proc Natl Acad Sci USA 1991; 88:2663-2667.

74. Tighe H, Friend PJ and Collier SJ. Delayed allograft rejection in

primates treated with anti-IL-2 receptor monoclonal antibody Campath-6. Transplantation 1988; 45:226-228.

75. Kupiec-Weglinski JW, Diamantstein T, Tilney NL and Strom TB. Therapy with monoclonal antibody to interleukin 2 receptor spares suppressor T cells and prevents or reverses acute allograft rejection in rats. Proc Natl Acad Sci USA 1986; 83:2624-2627.

76. Kirkman RL, Barrett LV, Galuton GN et al. Administration of an anti-interleukin 2 receptor monoclonal antibody prolongs allograft survival in mice. J Exp Med 1985; 162:358-362.

77. Tanaka K, Hancock WW, Osawa H et al. Mechanism of action of anti-IL-2R monoclonal antibodies: ART-18 prolongs cardiac allograft survival in rats by elimination of IL-2R⁺ mononuclear cells. J Immunol 1989; 143:2873-2879.

78. Kupiec-Weglinski JW, Tilney NL, Stunkel KG et al. Agonistic and antagonistic interactions of anti-interleukin 2 receptor monoclonal antibodies in rat recipients of cardiac allografts. Transplantation 1989; 47:11-16.

79. Wood MJA, Sloan DJ, Dallman MJ and Charlton HM. Specific tolerance to neural allografts induced with an antibody to the interleukin 2 receptor. J Exp Med 1993; 177:597-603.

80. Ueda H, Hancock WW, Cheung YC, Tanaka K, Kupiec-Weglinski JW and Tilney NL. Differential effects of interleukin 2 receptor-targeted therapy on heart and kidney allografts in rats. Depression of effectiveness of ART-18 monoclonal antibody treatment by uremia. Transplantation 1990; 49:1124-1129.

81. Tellides G, Dallman MJ, Kupiec-Weglinski JW, Diamantstein T and Morris PJ. Functional blocking of the interleukin-2 receptor (IL-2R) may be important in the efficacy of IL-2R antibody therapy. Transplant Proc 1987; 19:4231-4233.

82. Jacques Y, Paineau J, Chevalier S, Le Mauff B and Soulillou JP. A study on OX39, a murine anti-rat interleukin 2 receptor antibody:a report on receptor binding and effects on allograft survival. Transplant Int 1988; 1:58-63.

83. Ishizaka ST and Stutman O. Analysis by limiting dilution of interleukin-2 producing T cells in murine ontogeny. Eur J Immunol 1983; 13:936-942.

84. Malkovsky M, Medawar PB, Thatcher DR et al. Acquired immunological tolerance of foreign cells is impaired by recombinant interleukin 2 or vitamin A acetate. Proc Natl Acad Sci USA 1985; 82:536-538.

85. Malkovsky M and Medawar PB. Is immunological tolerance (nonresponsive) a consequence of interleukin 2 deficit during the recognition of antigen? Immunol Today 1984; 5:340-343.

86. Colizzi V. In vivo and in vitro administration of interleukin-2 containing preparation reverses T-cell unresponsiveness in *Mycobacterium bovis* BCG-infected mice. Infect Immun 1984; 45:25-28.

87. Dallman MJ, Shiho H, Page TH, Wood KJ and Morris PJ. Peri-

pheral tolerance to alloantigen results from altered regulation of the interleukin 2 pathway. J Exp Med 1991; 173:79-87.

88. Schwartz RH. A cell culture model for T lymphocyte clonal anergy. Science 1990; 248:1349-1356.

89. Kang SM, Beverly B, Tran AC, Brorson K, Schwartz RH and Lenardo MJ. Transactivation by AP-1 is a molecular target of T cell clonal anergy. Science 1992; 257:1134-1138.

90. Alters SE, Shizuru JA, Ackerman J, Grossman D, Seydl KB and Fathman CG. Anti-CD4 mediates clonal anergy during transplantation tolerance induction. J Exp Med 1991; 173:491-494.

91. Dallman MJ, Wood KJ, Hamano K et al. Cytokines and peripheral tolerance to alloantigen. Immunol Rev 1993; 133:5-18.

92. Boussiotis VA, Barber DL, Nakarai T et al. Prevention of T cell energy by signalling through the gamma c chain of the IL-2 receptor. Science 1994; 266:1039-1042.

93. Hahn HJ, Kuttler B, Kloting I, Dunger A, Besch W and Diamantstein T. Extended survival of MHC-identical allogeneic islet grafts in diabetic BB rats—the effect of an interleukin 2 receptor-targeted immunotherapy. Transplantation 1992; 54:555-558.

94. Cantarovich D, Le Mauff B, Hourmant M et al. Anti-interleukin 2 receptor monoclonal antibody in the treatment of ongoing acute rejection episodes of human kidney graft–a pilot study. Transplantation 1989; 47:454-457.

95. Carl S, Wiesel M, Daniel V and Staehler G. Effect of the anti-IL-2 receptor monoclonal antibody BT—563 in treatment of acute interstitial renal rejection. Transplant Proc 1995; 27:854.

96. Soulillou JP, Cantarovich D, Le Mauff B et al. Randomised controlled trial of a monoclonal antibody against the interleukin-2 receptor (33B3.1) as compared with rabbit antithymocyte globulin for prophylaxis against rejection of renal allografts. N Engl J Med 1990; 322:1175-1182.

97. Kriaa F, Hiesse C, Alard P et al. Prophylactic use of the anti-IL-2 receptor monoclonal antibody LO-Tact-1 in cadaveric renal transplantation:results of a randomized study. Transplant Proc 1993; 25:817-819.

98. Cantarovich D, Le Mauff B, Hourmant M et al. Prevention of acute rejection episodes with an anti-interleukin 2 receptor monoclonal antibody. I. Results after combined pancreas and kidney transplantation. Transplantation 1994; 57:198-203.

99. Hourmant M, Le Mauff B, Cantarovich D et al. Prevention of acute rejection episodes with an anti-interleukin 2 receptor monoclonal antibody. II. Results after a second kidney transplantation. Transplantation 1994; 57:204-207.

100. Kirkman RL, Shapiro ME, Carpenter CB et al. A randomised prospective trial of anti-Tac monoclonal antibody in human renal transplantation. Transplantation 1991; 51:107-113.

101. Amlot PL, Rawlings E, Fernando ON et al. Prolonged action of a

chimeric IL-2 receptor (CD25) monoclonal antibody used in cadaveric renal transplantation. Transplantation 1995; (in press)

102. Cantarovich D, Le Mauff B, Hourmant M et al. Prophylactic use of a monoclonal antibody (33B3.1) directed against interleukin 2 receptor following human renal transplantation. American Journal of Kidney Diseases 1988; XI:101-106.

103. Soulillou JP, Peyronnet P, Le Mauff B et al. Prevention of rejection of kidney transplants by monoclonal antibody directed against interleukin 2. Lancet 1987; 1:1339-1342.

104. van Gelder T, Kroes LCM, Mulder A, Gratama J and Weimar W. A living-related kidney donor as the source of a nearly fatal primary Epstein-Barr virus infection following transplantation. Transplantation 1994; 58:852-855.

105. Reding R, Vraux H, de Ville de Goyet J et al. Monoclonal antibodies in prophylactic immunosuppression after liver transplantation. A randomized controlled trial comparing OKT3 and anti-IL-2 receptor monoclonal antibody LO-Tact-1. Transplantation 1993; 55:534-541.

106. Otto G, Thies J, Kraus T et al. Monoclonal anti-CD25 for acute rejection after liver transplantation [letter]. Lancet 1991; 338:195

107. Neuhaus P, Bechstein WO, Blumhardt G et al. Comparison of quadruple immunosuppression after liver transplantation with ATG or IL-2 receptor antibody. Transplantation 1993; 55:1320-1327.

108. Herve P, Racadot E, Wendling D et al. Use of monoclonal antibodies in vivo as a therapeutic strategy for alloimmune or autoimmune reactivity: the Besancon experience. Immunol Rev 1992; 129:31-55.

109. Herbelin C, Stephan JL, Donadieu J et al. Treatment of steroid-resistant acute graft-versus-host disease with an anti-IL-2-receptor monoclonal antibody (BT 563) in children who received T cell-depleted, partially matched, related bone marrow transplants. Bone Marrow Transplantation 1994; 13:563-569.

110. Cuthbert RJ, Phillips GL, Barnett MJ et al. Anti-interleukin-2 receptor monoclonal antibody (BT 563) in the treatment of severe acute GVHD refractory to systemic corticosteroid therapy. Bone Marrow Transplantation 1992; 10:451-455.

111. Anasetti C, Hansen JA, Waldmann TA et al. Treatment of acute graft-versus-host disease with humanized anti-Tac:an antibody that binds to the interleukin-2 receptor. Blood 1994; 84:1320-1327.

112. Anasetti C, Martin PJ, Hansen JA et al. A phase I-II study evaluating the murine anti-IL-2 receptor antibody 2A3 for treatment of acute graft-versus-host disease. Transplantation 1990; 50:49-54.

113. Ferrant A, Latinne D, Bazin H et al. Prophylaxis of graft-versus-host disease in identical sibling donor BMT by anti-IL-2 receptor monoclonal antibody LO-Tact-1. Blood 1995; (in press)

114. Blaise D, Olive D, Michallet M et al. Impairment of leukemia-free survival by addition of interleukin-2-receptor antibody to standard

graft-versus-host-prophylaxis. Lancet 1995; 345:1144-46.

115. Anasetti C, Martin PJ, Storb R et al. Prophylaxis of graft-versus-host disease by administration of the murine anti-IL-2 receptor antibody 2A3. Bone Marrow Transplantation 1991; 7:375-381.

116. Laufer G, Kukutschki W, Haan A et al. Prospective randomised trial of antithymocyte globulin vs. monoclonal IL-2 receptor antibody as early immunoprophylaxis after cardiac transplantation. 1993. (UnPub)

117. van Gelder T, Balk AH, Mochtar B and Weimar W. Reversal of graft rejection with monoclonal anti-interleukin-2 receptor [letter]. Lancet 1992; 339:873.

118. Janszen M, Buck D, Maino VC. Functional and molecular properties of CD25 monoclonal antibodies. Keukocyte Typing IV, ed Knapp W, Dorken B, Gilks WR et al. Oxford:Oxford University Press 1989; 403.

119. Wong JT, Schott E, Sabga EM, Kielpinski GG and Colvin RB. Immunogenic epitopes of the p55 chain of the IL-2 receptor. Transplantation 1990; 49:587-596.

120. Friend PJ, Tighe H, Waldmann H et al. Monoclonal antibodies that recognise activated human lymphocytes–experimental and clinical studies. Transplant Proc 1988; XX:265-266.

121. Rose B, Gillespie A, Wunderlich D et al. A chimeric mouse/human anti-IL-2 receptor antibody with enhanced biological activities. Mol Immunol 1992; 29:131-144.

122. Vandevyver C, Steukers M, Lambrechts J, Heyligen H and Raus J. Development and functional characterization of a murine/human chimeric antibody with specificity for the human interleukin-2 receptor. Mol Immunol 1993; 30:865-876.

123. Kaluza B, Lenz H, Russmann E et al. Synthesis and functional characterization of a recombinant monoclonal antibody directed against the alpha-chain of the human interleukin-2 receptor. Gene 1991; 107:297-305.

124. Weissenhorn W, Scheuer W, Kaluza B et al. Combinatorial functions of two chimeric antibodies directed to human CD4 and one directed to the alpha-chain of the human interleukin-2 receptor. Gene 1992; 121:271-278.

125. Queen C, Schneider WP, Selick HE et al. A humanised antibody that binds to the interleukin 2 receptor. Proc Natl Acad Sci USA 1989; 86:10029.

126. Nakatani T, Lone YC, Yamakawa J et al. Humanization of mouse anti-human IL-2 receptor antibody B-B10. Protein Engineering 1994; 7:435-443.

127. Kaluza B, Betzl G, Shao H, Diamantstein T and Weidle UH. A general method for chimerization of monoclonal antibodies by inverse polymerase chain reaction which conserves authentic N-terminal sequences. Gene 1992; 122:321-328.

128. Hakimi J, Ha VC, Lin P et al. Humanised Mikβ1, a humanised

antibody to the IL-2 receptor β-chain that acts synergistically with humanised anti-TAC. J Immunol 1993; 151:1075-1085.

129. Kelley VE, Bacha P, Pankewycz OG, Nichols JC, Murphy JR and Strom TB. Interleukin 2-diptheria toxin fusion protein can abolish cell-mediated immunity in vivo. Proc Natl Acad Sci USA 1988; 85:3980-3984.

130. Kirkman RL, Bacha P, Barrett LV, Forte SE, Murphy JR and Strom TB. Prolongation of cardiac allograft survival in murine recipients treated with a diptheria toxin-related interleukin-2 fusion protein. Transplantation 1989; 47:327-330.

131. LeMaistre CF, Meneghetti CM, Rosenblum MG et al. Phase I trial of an interleukin-2 (IL-2) fusion toxin (DAB$_{486}$) in haematological malignancies expressing the IL-2 receptor. Blood 1992; 79:2547-2554.

132. Vie H, Gauthier T, Breathnach R et al. Human fusion proteins between interleukin 2 and IgM heavy chain are cytotoxic for cells expressing the interleukin 2 receptor. Proc Natl Acad Sci USA 1992; 89:11337-11341.

133. Takeshita T, Goto Y, Tada K, Nagata K, Asao H and Sugamura K. Monoclonal antibody defining a molecule possibly identical to the p75 subunit of interleukin 2 receptor. J Exp Med 1989; 169:1323-1332.

134. Nakamura Y, Inamoto T, Sugie K et al. Mitogenicity and down-regulation of high-affinity interleukin 2 receptor by YTA-1 and YTA-2 monoclonal antibodies that recognise 75-kDa molecules on human large granular lymphocytes. Proc Natl Acad Sci USA 1989; 86:1318-1322.

135. Ohbo K, Takeshita T, Asao H et al. Monoclonal antibodies defining distinct epitopes of the human IL-2 receptor beta chain and their differential effects on IL-2 responses. J Immunol Methods 1991; 142:61-72.

136. Francois C, Boeffard F, Kaluza B, Weidle UH and Jacques Y. Construction of a bispecific antibody reacting with the alpha-and beta-chains of the human IL-2 receptor. High affinity cross-linking and high anti-proliferative efficiency. J Immunol 1993; 150:4610-4619.

137. Gnarra JR, Otani H, Wang MG, McBride OW, Sharon M and Leonard WJ. Human interleukin 2 receptor beta-chain gene:chromosomal localization and identification of 5' regulatory sequences. Proc Natl Acad Sci USA 1990; 87:3440-3444.

138. Shibuya H, Yoneyama M, Nakamura Y et al. The human interleukin-2 receptor β chain gene:genomic organisation, promoter analysis and chromosomal assignment. Nucleic Acids Research 1990; 18:3697-3703.

139. Arima N, Karnio M, Imada K et al. Pseudo-high affinity interleukin 2 (IL-2) receptor lacks the third component that is essential

for functional IL-2 binding and signaling. J Exp Med 1992; 176:1265-1272.

140. Cosman D, Lyman SD, Idzerda RL et al. A new cytokine receptor superfamily. Trends in Biochemical Science 1990; 15:265-269.

141. Ohashi Y, Takeshita T, Nagata K, Mori S and Sugamura K. Differential expression of the IL-2 receptor subunits, p55 and p75 on various populations of primary peripheral blood mononuclear cells. J Immunol 1989; 143:3548-3555.

142. Yagita H, Nakata M, Azuma A et al. Activation of peripheral blood T cells via the p75 interleukin 2 receptor. J Exp Med 1989; 170:1445-1450.

143. Djeu JY, Liu JH, Wei S et al. Function associated with IL-2 receptor-b on human neutrophils. Mechanism of activation of antifungal activity against *Candida albicans* by IL-2. J Immunol 1993; 150:960-970.

144. Ferrara JLM, Marion A, McIntyre JF, Murphy GF and Burakoff SJ. Amelioration of acute graft vs host disease due to minor histocompatibility antigens by in vivo administration of anti-interleukin 2 receptor antibody. J Immunol 1986; 137:1874-1877.

145. Volk H, Brocke S, Osawa H and Diamantstein T. Effects of in-vivo administration of a monoclonal antibody specific for the interleukin-2 receptor on the acute graft-versus-host reaction in mice. Clin Exp Immunol 1986; 66:126-131.

146. Kupiec-Weglinski JW, Sablinski T, Hancock WW, Di Stefano R, Mariani G and Tilney NL. Modulation of accelerated rejection of cardiac allografts in sensitized rats by anti-interleukin 2 receptor monoclonal antibody and cyclosporine therapy. Transplantation 1991; 51:300-305.

147. Ueda H, Hancock WW, Cheung Y, Diamantstein T, Tilney NL and Kupiec-Weglinski JW. The mechanism of synergistic interaction between anti-interleukin 2 receptor monoclonal antibody and cyclosporine therapy in rat recipients of organ allografts. Transplantation 1990; 50:545-550.

148. Hancock WW, DiStefano R, Braun P, Schweizer RT, Tilney NL and Kupiec-Weglinski JW. Cyclosporine and anti-interleukin 2 receptor monoclonal antibody therapy suppress accelerated rejection of rat cardiac allografts through different effector mechanisms. Transplantation 1990; 49:416-421.

149. van Gelder T, Zietse R, Yzermans JNM, Vaessen LMB, Mulder AH and Weimar W. Monoclonal anti-IL-2 receptor antibody (BT563) prevents early rejection after kidney transplantation. A double blind, placebo controlled trial. Transplant Proc 1995; (in press).

150. Hiesse C, Kriaa F, Alard P et al. Prophylactic use of the IL-2 receptor-specific monoclonal antibody LO-Tact-1 with cyclosporin A and steroids in renal transplantation. Transplant Int 1992; 5:S444-S447.

151. Friend PJ, Waldmann H, Cobbold S et al. The anti-IL-2 receptor monoclonal antibody YTH-906 in liver transplantation. Transplant Proc 1991; 23:1390-1392.
152. Herve P, Wijdenes J, Bergerat JP et al. Treatment of corticosteroid resistant acute-graft-versus-host disease by in vivo administration of anti-interleukin-2 receptor monoclonal antibody (B-B10). Blood 1990; 75:1017-1023.
153. Tiley C, Powles R, Teo CP, Treleaven J, Findlay M and Hewetson M. Treatment of acute graft versus host disease with a murine monoclonal antibody to the IL-2 receptor. Bone Marrow Transplantation 1991; 7 Suppl 2:151
154. Belanger C, Esperou-Bourdeau H, Bordigoni P et al. Use of an anti-interleukin-2 receptor monoclonal antibody for GVHD prophylaxis in unrelated donor BMT. Bone Marrow Transplantation 1993; 11:293-297.
155. Burdach S, Mauz C, Hanenberg H et al. Prevention of acute and chronic graft versus host disease (GVHD) with prolonged p55 IL2 receptor antibody therapy in bone marrow transplant recipients at high risk for GVHD. Blood 1995; (in press)
156. Beliard R. Selection d'un anticorps monoclonal anti-recepteur de l'interleukine-2 humaine en vue d'une utilisation therapeutique. 1991; 60-76.(Abstract)
157. Engert A, Martin G, Amlot PL, Wijdenes J, Diehl V and Thorpe PE. Immunotoxins constructed with anti-CD25 monoclonal antibodies and deglycosylated ricin A-chain have potent anti-tumour effects against human Hodgkin cells in vitro and solid Hodgkin tumours in mice. Int J Cancer 1991; 49:450-456.

THE USE OF OKT3 IN CLINICAL TRANSPLANTATION

Daniel Abramowicz and Michel Goldman

INTRODUCTION

OKT3 is a murine monoclonal antibody of the IgG2a isotype recognizing the ε chain of the CD3 complex, a series of proteins tightly linked to the individual T-cell receptor present on all mature T cells.[1,2] OKT3 has been produced by immunization of mice with human T cells in 1979.[1] The discovery that OKT3 blocked in vitro the lytic activity of cytotoxic T cells[3,4] led to its use in renal allograft rejection,[5] even before the molecular structure recognized on T lymphocytes was identified. Since then, extensive data have shown that OKT3 is probably the most potent drug available to treat rejection of organ allografts.[6-11] In addition, as avoidance of rejection in the early post-transplant period might be a determining factor in the achievement of successful long-term allograft survival, OKT3 has been evaluated as an inductive agent in renal transplantation.[6-12] In this review, we first define the mechanisms of action of OKT3. We then describe the main studies that established its efficacy both for the treatment and the prevention of renal allograft rejection. Finally, we discuss its main side effects and strategies to prevent them.

Monoclonal Antibodies in Transplantation, edited by Lucienne Chatenoud. © 1995 R.G. Landes Company.

MECHANISMS OF ACTION OF OKT3

DEPLETION

Within minutes after injection of OKT3, T cells disappear from the circulation.[5,13-14] The basis of this effect has yet to be fully elucidated, but several mechanisms might be operative. First, OKT3 upregulates adhesion molecules on both T cells and endothelial cells. T cells display increased LFA-1 expression after stimulation by OKT3,[15] while upregulation of VCAM-1, the counter receptor for VLA-4, is found on endothelial cells from mice injected with activating anti-CD3 antibodies.[16] Obviously, both processes will promote adhesion of T cells to vascular endothelium. Second, opsonisation of T cells probably also plays a role in T-cell depletion. Indeed, OKT3 activates human complement in vivo, and T cells bearing C3b fragments can be detected after incubation with OKT3 in vitro.[17] Furthermore, interactions between OKT3-coated T cells and monocytes-macrophages bearing FcγRI, the human Fc receptor which binds murine IgG2a antibodies, will also lead to opsonisation. T-cell death might also occur through induction of apoptosis[18] or by redirected T-cell lysis,[19] a process which occurs when OKT3 bridges a T cell—either CD4 or CD8—with a cytotoxic CD8 cell. While further experiments are needed to clarify the main mechanisms responsible for the rapid disappearance of T cells from blood, data obtained in mouse and man suggest that both redistribution and lysis do occur after anti-CD3 administration.

Table 4.1. Immunosuppressive effects of anti-CD3/TCR antibodies

1. Depletion of circulating T cells
   a. Redistribution
      Increased expression of LFA-1 on T cells/VCAM-1 on endothelial cells
   b. Lysis/death
      1. Complement
      2. Apoptosis
      3. Redirected lysis by CTL
      4. Opsonisation / phagocytosis
2. Modulation of CD3/TCR complex
3. Functional blockade of CD3/TCR complex
4. Induction of T cell unresponsiveness
   a. No proliferation to IL-2
   b. Inhibition of IL-2 production
   c. Desensitisation of CD3/TCR complex
5. Induction of tolerance to alloantigens ?

MODULATION

While virtually no T cells are detectable in the peripheral blood during the first days of OKT3 therapy, T cells gradually reappear subsequently, but with CD3 modulated from their cell membrane.[13,14] Thus, CD2+ cells, both of the CD4 and CD8 phenotype circulate, but they lack membrane expression of the T-cell receptor-CD3 complex. These modulated T cells are unable to recognize alloantigens, and have been shown to be non-functionnal in vitro.

BLOCKADE

The ability of OKT3 to inhibit the lysis mediated by activated cytotoxic T cells has been the basis for its initial use in allograft rejection. It is postulated that by coating CD3 antigens, OKT3 blocks the interaction between the T-cell receptor and its target by steric hindrance, thereby preventing cell activation.[3-4,20-22]

The remarkable clinical efficacy of OKT3 probably stems from its multiple and probably synergistic immunosuppressive effects—depletion, modulation and blockade. For instance, modulation of the T-cell receptor/CD3 complex should markedly reduce the amounts of OKT3 necessary to block residual free TCR-CD3. In support of this idea, very high OKT3 concentrations are needed to block cytotoxic T cells in experimental settings not allowing for modulation to occur.[3-4]

Thus, immunosuppression during the period of OKT3 administration certainly results from this immunosuppressive umbrella that prevents contact between T cells and alloantigens. Moreover, several experiments have shown that anti-CD3/TCR antibodies may render the T cells anergic and favor the induction of long-lasting tolerance to alloantigens.

INDUCTION OF T-CELL UNRESPONSIVENESS

The following defects in T-cell function have been observed after multivalent cross-linking of the CD3/TCR complex by MoAbs.

Unresponsiveness to IL-2

Activation of T cells with high concentrations of immobilized anti-CD3 antibodies will lead to inability to proliferate in the presence of IL-2, despite adequate induction of membrane IL-2 receptor expression.[23-25] Addition of cyclosporine A does not prevent IL-2 unresponsiveness.[25]

Inhibition of IL-2 production

When T-cell activation occurs in the absence of costimulatory signals, such as those provided by engagement of the CD28 molecule, inability to produce IL-2 may ensue even when adequate stimulation is then provided.[26-27] Cyclosporine A will prevent induction of this particular type of anergy, probably because it is an active phenomenon dependent on calcium influx. Of interest, the limited T-cell activation and calcium flux associated with non-mitogenic anti-CD3 IgM antibodies is sufficient to induce this phenomenon.[28]

Defective TCR signal transduction following T-cell activation

Stimulation of T-cell clones and hybridomas through the CD3/TCR complex results in IL-2 production and proliferation. However, this also leads to subsequent long-term inability to produce IL-2 after stimulation trough the CD3/TCR complex.[29-30] Recent experiments indicate that the early steps consecutive to T-cell receptor cross-linking, such as calcium influx, are deficient in hyporesponsive cells. Stimuli that bypass the TCR/CD3 complex, such as ionomycin together with phorbol esters, remain efficient.[30] Whether similar uncoupling/desensitisation of the TCR from the intracellular activation machinery also occurs in normal T-cell populations remains to be elucidated.

Some of these and possibly other as yet unidentified mechanisms might be involved in the ability of anti-CD3 antibodies to induce anergy in normal T cells.[31-31] One study specifically addressed the effect of anti-CD3 antibodies on the priming of human T cells to alloantigens in vitro.[33] In these experiments, addition of anti-CD3 antibodies to a primary mixed lymphocyte culture between peripheral blood mononuclear cells and allogeneic stimulators resulted in specific anergy, as shown by absence of proliferation in a subsequent culture with the priming but not with third-party alloantigens. These results have been extended to in vivo situations, where anti-TCR/CD3 antibodies have been shown to induce long-term specific tolerance to allografts in rodents.[34-37] Obviously, anti-TCR/CD3 antibodies have the potential to lead to transplantation tolerance.

Future research will focus on the following questions: 1) Is T-cell activation necessary for subsequent immunosuppression? 2) If yes, then will discrete steps in T-cell activation suffice to ensure optimal immunosuppression, or will full activation as seen with OKT3 be required? 3) Will the characteristics of the anti-CD3/ TCR MoAbs for efficient treatment of rejection and prophylaxis be the same? Most importantly, strategies will have to be developed to increase the tolerogenic effects of anti-TCR/CD3 antibodies. Possible synergy with other drugs that inhibit T-cell function such as cyclosporine or rapamycin, with reagents that block costimulatory molecules, or with infusion of donor hematopoietic cells deserves to be investigated.

STUDIES IN GRAFT REJECTION

OKT3 vs glucocorticosteroids for first-line rejection treatment

Basal immunosuppression without cyclosporine A

Initial studies used doses of OKT3 of 1 or 2 mg in patients with renal allograft rejection.[5] While initial rejection reversal occurred, only low OKT3 serum levels were achieved and rejection rapidly recurred. This problem could be alleviated by increasing OKT3 dose to 5 mg/day.[5] These pioneer observations set the stage for the Ortho multicenter study comparing OKT3 with high-dose steroids as first-line treatment of renal rejection episodes[38] (Table 4.2). 62 patients received OKT3, at a dose of 5 mg/day, for 14 days together with azathioprine and low-dose steroids, and were compared to 60 patients who received high-dose steroids (500 mg for 3 days followed by a progressive taper). Reversal of rejection was more frequent in the OKT3 group (94% vs 75% in the steroid group, p = 0.009). Importantly, this allowed for an improved graft survival at 1 year in OKT3 patients (62% vs 45% in the steroid group, p = 0.029). It must be noted that equine antithymocyte globulin and not OKT3 was used for rescue treatment of resistant rejections in the steroid group. The incidence of recurrent rejection after therapy was similar in both groups (66% in OKT3 vs 73% in the steroid group).

Basal immunosuppression including cyclosporine A

While cyclosporine A was not part of basal immunosuppression in the Ortho study, two retrospective studies have shown a higher efficiency of OKT3 as first-line therapy of acute renal graft rejection as compared to steroids in patients receiving cyclosporin A as maintenance immunosuppression. In the first study (39), rejection was reversed by OKT3 in 28/34 patients (82%) as compared to 34/54 patients treated with steroids (63%) (p = 0.06) (Table 4.2). Cyclosporine A was maintained at least at half-doses during rejection therapy. Resistant rejections were treated with steroids in OKT3 patients and with OKT3 in steroid patients, with reversal achieved in 3/5 vs 12/18 patients respectively (p = ns). Thus, with primary and rescue treatments combined, the reversal rate was around 90% in both groups. Three-months graft survival was also similar in both groups (74%).

In the second study, in which CsA was begun after induction therapy with ALG, treatment of the first kidney rejection episode with OKT3 resulted in graft survival at 1 and 2 years 11% and 20% greater respectively than in patients treated with steroids.[40] Cyclosporine A was maintained during rejection therapy as long as serum creatinine concentration remained below 3.5 mg/dl. Of importance, first cadaver transplant recipients benefited particularly from OKT3 therapy (graft survival at 2 years: 87% vs 54% in steroid group, p = 0.033) (Table 4.2). However, only low doses of steroids were used to treat rejection (oral prednisone 2 mg/kg/day tapered to 0.2 mg/kg by day 14), so that it is unclear whether the superiority of OKT3 in this study is related to its intrinsic efficacy or to suboptimal doses of steroids.

Concern has been raised that rejection treatment with OKT3 might lead to increased incidence of subsequent rejection[41] but this has not been observed in the 3 above-mentioned studies. Several other open, retrospective studies have indicated that reversal of graft rejection occurs in 80 to 90% of patients treated with OKT3 (Table 4.2).[42]

Thus, the possibility that in the cyclosporine era first-line therapy with OKT3 rather than with steroids would lead to improved long-term kidney graft survival remains open, and clearly warrants further evaluation (see below).

Table 4.2. First-line treatment of renal allograft rejection: comparison between OKT3 and high-dose steroids.

Study	Design	Cyclosporine A use		Variable	OKT3	Steroids	P
		Before rejection	During rejection				
Ortho	Prospective randomized	No	No	N° of patients	62	60	–
				Rejection reversal	94%	75%	0.009
				Graft survival (1 year)	62%	45%	0.029
Deierhoi	Retrospective	Yes	Yes	N° of patients	34	54	–
				Rejection reversal	82%	63%	0.06
				Graft survival (3 months)	74%	74%	NS
Tesi	Retrospective	Yes	Yes	N° of patients[A]	39	38	–
				Graft survival (2 years)	87%	54%	0.033

[A] Recipients of first cadaveric grafts

OKT3 as second or third line treatment

Open trials

Over the past years, it has become clear from numerous open, uncontrolled trials that OKT3 could reverse renal rejection episodes resistant to treatment with steroids (second-line therapy).[42] In this setting, rejection reversal with OKT3 ranged between 50 to 100% and allowed graft survival at one year to reach values between 40 and 74%.[43] Good results have also been observed when OKT3 was used to treat rejection episodes resistant to both steroids and polyclonal anti-lymphocyte antibodies. Whether this is related to intrinsic properties of OKT3 or just from prolonged and profound immunosuppression is unknown. In addition, this heavy immunosuppression carries the risk of increased infectious episodes and lymphomas (see below).

The overall good rejection reversal rate with OKT3 as rescue therapy, combined with the cost and side effects of OKT3, led many transplant centers to try steroids for rejection first. This therapy is expected to reverse 70% of acute episodes, OKT3 being spared for cases of corticoresistance. Both strategies—OKT3 as first line therapy, or steroids followed by OKT3 for corticoresistant rejections—are expected to reverse about 90% of rejection episodes. However, rejection reversal is a short-term outcome, and the critical issue of long-term graft survival in the cyclosporine era still needs to be properly addressed. Indeed, the following questions remain open in patients taking cyclosporine A: 1) Does primary therapy of renal graft rejection with OKT3 improve long-term graft survival as compared to high-dose steroids? 2) Is any possible increase in graft survival limited to high-risk recipients, such as re-transplant or immunized patients, or those receiving a poorly HLA-matched kidney? 3) Is primary therapy of rejection with OKT3 still be valuable in patients who received prophylaxis with poly- or monoclonal antilymphocyte agents? Given the large numbers of patients required to demonstrate that a medically important improvement such as a 10% increase in graft survival is statistically significant, it is likely that answers, if any, will come from analysis of data from the large transplant registries rather than from prospective studies.

Comparison with polyclonal antilymphocyte antibodies

Several trials compared OKT3 with polyclonal antilymphocyte preparations for treatment of steroid-resistant rejections. Hesse observed improved function after treatment with ALG (horse Lymphoglobuline from Institut Mérieux, France) in 8/10 patients and in 10/11 after OKT3 therapy.[44] In another study comparing OKT3 to ATG (rabbit thymoglobuline from Mérieux), the number of graft failures was similar in both groups (4/26 in OKT3 vs 11/32 in ATG patients), but graft survival was higher at 2 years in OKT3 patients (88% vs 63%, p = 0.05).[45] Finally, a rabbit ATG preparation (Fresenius) reversed steroid-resistant rejection in 5/9 patients as compared with 5/8 with OKT3.[46] Although the number of patients enrolled in these studies was often limited, both polyclonal anti-lymphocyte agents and OKT3 appear to be as efficient in treating cortico-resistant renal rejection episodes.

OKT3 in vascular rejection

Vascular injury during rejection, characterized by endothelial swelling and infiltration of vessel wall by mononuclear cell infiltrates, is known to be a pejorative factor in the outcome of rejection. It is now recognized that T cells play a major role in the initiation of vascular lesions like they do in acute cellular, interstitial rejection. OKT3 was first shown to reverse steroid-resistant, predominantly vascular acute rejection in 3 patients.[47] This was confirmed in a later study that showed that OKT3 reversed 86% of mixed vascular and cellular rejection as compared to 91% of cellular episodes, although 1-year graft survival was lower in patients with vascular lesions vs those with purely cellular rejection (58% vs 75%, p = 0.08).[48] The efficiency of OKT3 in this setting might seem paradoxical in view of its ability to activate endothelial cells and to promote procoagulant activities (**see below**). It might be that in vascular rejection, OKT3 has both beneficial effects—by clearing the T-cell infiltrate—as well as detrimental effects, by promoting intravascular thromboses. That such a delicate balance exists is supported by the inefficiency of OKT3 in vascular rejections once intraglomerular thromboses had occurred.[49]

STUDIES ON OKT3 PROPHYLAXIS

OKT3 versus cyclosporinee for induction of immunosuppression

The efficacy of OKT3 in the treatment of rejection episodes led to its use as prophylaxis in cadaveric kidney transplantation. The rationale was that 1) the most potent immunosuppressive agent should be used in the immediate post-operative period, in the hope to better prevent early rejection and 2) the introduction of cyclosporine A could then be delayed, avoiding early nephrotoxicity.

Two randomized and two nonrandomized trials have demonstrated that OKT3 induction therapy is more effective than triple-drug therapy in terms of length of time until the onset of rejections, percentage of patients with rejections, and graft survival[50-53] (Table 4.3). The two randomized studies performed in Belgium[52] and in the USA[53] utilized a triple-drug regimen consisting of azathioprine, steroids, and either OKT3 or cyclosporine A. Patients treated with OKT3 received 5 mg/day for 7 to 21 days (mean 14 days) with the addition of cyclosporine on the last 3 to 4 days. The percentage of patients with rejection episodes during follow-up was significantly lower with OKT3 induction in comparison to cyclosporine induction in all studies reporting this statistic $(0.05 > P > 0.001)$ (Table 4.3). A delay in time to rejection with prophylactic OKT3 therapy was evidenced in all studies in which these times were reported. In the Belgian randomized trial, the mean interval to first rejection episode in the course of the first three post-transplant months was 23.1 days in OKT3 patients versus 11.3 in cyclosporinee patients $(P < 0.001)$. Interestingly, in that study a higher number of rejection episodes were found to be corticosensitive in OKT3 patients (52 out of 61 rejection episodes (85%) vs. 57 out of 81 (70%) in cyclosporinee patients, $P = 0.045$). In the U.S. randomized trial, the median number of days to first rejection was 45.5 in the OKT3-treatment group (54 patients) compared to 8.0 days in the cyclosporinee-treated patients (67 patients) $(P = 0.001)$. Similarly in a nonrandomized study, the median time to first rejection was 23.5 days in the OKT3-treated group compared to 11 days in the cyclosporinee-treated patients $(P < 0.05)$. The other non-randomized study also showed a considerably longer time to rejection in OKT3 as compared to cyclosporinee-treated patients. However, the difference did not reach significance, probably because of the small sample size.

Table 4.3. Induction of immunosuppression with OKT3 in cadaveric renal transplants: comparison to early cyclosporine in triple-drug regimens with azathioprine and corticosteroids

Study	OKT3				Cyclosporine			
	N	Percent patients with rejection episodes (follow-up)	Days to initial rejection episode	Percent graft survival (follow-up)	N	Percent patients with rejection episodes (follow-up)	Days to initial rejection episode	Percent graft survival (follow-up)
Randomized Studies								
Abramowicz et al. 1992(3)	56	62[a] (18 m)	23.1[b]	88 (1 y) 84 (3 y)	52	77 (18 m)	11.3	77 (1 y) 75 (3 y)
Norman et al. 1993(4)	105	51[c] (1 y)	45.5[d] (median)	90 (1 y) 84 (2 y) 73 (5 y)	102	67 (1 y)	8.0 (median)	82 (1 y) 75 (2 y) 64 (5 y)
Nonrandomized Studies								
Benvenisty et al. 1990(1)	34 (ATN)	44[e] (22.6±2.0 m)[f]	23.5[e] (median)	80[e] (1 y) 74 (2 y)	40	82 (40.7±2.7 m)[f]	11.0 (median)	55 (1 y) 47 (2 y)
Dafoe et al. 1991(5)	38 (+AGXM) 32 (−AGXM)[g]	44 (3 m) 44 (3 m)	35 (mean) 22 (mean)	82 (1 y) 78 (1 y)	10 (+AGXM) 32 (−AGXM)[g]	70 (3 m) 73 (3 m)[h]	13 (mean) 13 (mean)	70 (1 y) 81 (1 y)

AGXM=antiglobulin crossmatch; ATN=acute tubular necrosis; NR=not reported; m=month; y=year.
[a] Significantly different from cyclosporine (p=0.04).
[b] Significantly different from cyclosporine in the course of the first three months (p < 0.001).
[c] Significantly different from cyclosporine (p=0.032).
[d] Significantly different from cyclosporine (p=0.001).
[e] Significantly different from cyclosporine (p < 0.05).
[f] Mean±standard deviation.
[g] Patients with immediate function received cyclosporine while those requiring dialysis received OKT3.
[h] Primary nonfunction grafts excluded.

A remarkably similar trend towards improved overall graft survival after OKT3 induction was observed in the two randomized trials: 84% at 2 years in the USA and 83% at 3 years in Belgium in OKT3 patients as compared to 75% in both trials for cyclosporine patients (Table 4.3).

Interest of OKT3 induction in high-risk recipients

OKT3 induction could be especially beneficial in high-risk recipients, such as those with delayed graft function. Thus, in a non-randomized study in patients with acute tubular necrosis (ATN), the 80% 1-year survival obtained with OKT3 induction therapy was significantly higher than the 55% survival reported in historical controls receiving cyclosporinee[50] (P < 0.05) (Table 4.3). Furthermore, the mean length of allograft non-function was shorter (9.4 vs 14.9 days, P < 0.05), and the mean number of inpatient hospital days was lower (23.9 vs 33.2, P < 0.05) for the OKT3-induction group. Similarly, in a non-comparative study of 25 patients with ATN who received OKT3 induction therapy, a 1-year graft survival of 84% (in comparison to a previous 63% 1-year graft survival in patients with ATN), a median duration of delayed graft function of 10 days, and a mean hospital stay of 21 days were observed.[54] In one additional non-randomized comparative study, similar one-year graft survival was observed in patients with ATN who were given OKT3 (78%) as compared to those with functioning grafts who received cyclosporinee (81%).[51]

Retransplant or immunized patients also experience substantial benefits from OKT3 induction. An open clinical trial of prophylactic treatment with OKT3 in high-risk patients was conducted in 27 patients who had received multiple transplants and/or had panel reactive antibody (PRA) levels greater than 50%. OKT3 was part of a quadruple-drug immunosuppressive regimen consisting of azathioprine, prednisone, and cyclosporinee (cyclosporinee was initiated when serum creatinine fell to below 4 mg/dL). Patients receiving OKT3 in this study showed a 1-year graft survival of 70% compared to a rate of 50% in a historical set of similar patients.[55]

A recent report from the UNOS Scientific Renal Transplant Registry analyzing data of 23.000 cadaveric renal transplants confirms the superiority of OKT3 induction over cyclosporine in recipient and donor high-risk groups. Indeed, significant and clinically meaningful 5 to 10% improvement in 1-year graft survival occurred in retransplant, sensitized, and diabetic recipients, as well as in those with ATN. In addition, recipients from high-risk donors—those with cerebro-vascular accidents or over 55 years of age—also enjoyed similar increase in graft survival.[56]

Although the above-mentioned studies strongly suggested the interest of OKT3 prophylaxis in high-risk groups, none of them was prospective or randomized. As the immunosuppressive regimen used in the Belgian and U.S. multicenter study was nearly identical (see above), we recently merged the databases from these two studies after having updated the patient data.[57] The demographic characteristics of the 296 patients (152 in the OKT3 group and 144 in the CsA group) were not different between both groups. There were 10 deaths in OKT3 vs 9 in CsA patients (P = NS). Forty-nine grafts were lost (34%) in CsA patients vs 42 (27.6 %) in OKT3 patients (P = 0.233). Rejection was the main cause of graft loss in both CsA and OKT3 groups (45 vs 32, P = 0.046). Actuarial graft survival, taking into account all causes of graft losses, was higher in OKT3 patients (at 2 years, 83.6% in OKT3 vs 73.6% in CsA patients, P = 0.03; at 5 years, 71.2% in OKT3 vs 65% in CsA patients, P = 0.152).

In order to better delineate the subsets of patients in whom OKT3 prophylaxis would be most beneficial, we first analyzed 5-years graft survival in relation to HLA-DR matching. While CsA patients with 2 HLA-DR mismatches (N = 26) had lower graft survival than those with 0 or 1 mismatch (N = 118) (56% vs 67%), this was not the case in OKT3 patients (N = 37 with 2 and 115 with 0 or 1 HLA-DR mismatches; graft survival at 5 y: 73 vs 71%, P = NS). Thus, graft survival in OKT3 patients with 2 HLA-DR mismatches was much higher than in CsA patients with 2 mismatches (73 vs 56%). This comparison did not reach significance (P = 0.163) probably because of the low number of patients receiving kidneys poorly matched at the HLA-DR locus in this trial.

We next analyzed graft survival in recipients of kidneys with cold ischemia either shorter or longer than 24 h. While CsA recipients of kidneys with long cold ischemia (N = 74) had significantly lower graft survival than those with short ischemia (N = 70) (at 2 y: 68 vs 92%; at 5 y: 56 vs 74%, P = 0.015), this was not the case in OKT3 patients (N = 71 with long cold ischemia and

81 with short ischemia; at 2 y: 88 vs 89%; at 5 y: 66 vs 76%, P = NS). Moreover, graft survival in OKT3 recipients with prolonged ischemia approaches that in CsA recipients with short ischemia, and was much higher than in CsA patients with long ischemia (P = 0.06).

Finally, we divided patients in 2 groups taking into account both the duration of cold ischemia and the number of HLA-DR mismatches. Patients with cold ischemia time less than 24 h and 0 or 1 HLA-DR mismatch were defined as low-risk patients, while all the others (cold ischemia > 24 h and/or 2 HLA-DR mismatches) were considered as high-risk patients. While graft survival was higher in low-risk (N = 58) than in high-risk (N = 86) CsA patients (at 5 y: 72 vs 61%, P = 0.037), it was similar for both risk groups in OKT3 patients (59 low and 93 high-risk patients; at 5 y: 73 vs 71%, P = NS). At 5 y in high-risk patients, OKT3 prophylaxis allowed for a significant 10% improvement in long-term graft survival as compared to CsA (71 vs 61%, P = 0.033).

Two conclusions can be drawn from this study. First, OKT3 prophylaxis does not improve long-term graft survival as compared to CsA in cadaveric kidney graft recipients at low risk for rejection. Second, OKT3 prophylaxis allowed high-risk recipients to achieve 5-year graft survival rate similar to those of low-risk recipients. Importantly, this resulted in a significant 10% increase in long-term kidney graft survival as compared to CsA-treated high-risk patients.

It is thus clear that prophylaxis with OKT3 results in clinically important improvement in long-term graft survival in patients at high immunological risk. On biological grounds, it appears that the situations in which OKT3 significantly improves graft survival are associated with increased alloreactive responses. This could be related to enhanced immunogenicity of the graft as in case of poor HLA matching or prolonged ischemia, or to priming of the recipient as in immunized or retransplant patients. In these settings, the ability of OKT3 to block T-cell function might be of particular interest as it would let time for the early ischemic injury and inflammatory reactions consecutive to organ procurement to subside. This would result in reduced graft immunogenicity when T cells reappear at the end of OKT3 administration, possibly accounting for the long-term benefits of this therapy.

Table 4.4. Results of studies comparing induction of immunosuppression with either OKT3 or polyclonal antibodies in renal transplants using drug regimens that included azathioprine, corticosteroids, and cyclosporine

Study	Type of study	OKT3			Polyclonal antibodies		
		N (Type of graft)	Percent patients with rejection episodes (follow-up)	Percent graft survival (follow-up)	N (Type of graft)	Percent patients with rejection episodes (follow-up)	Percent graft survival (follow-up)
Broyer et al 1993	Randomized	77 (Kidney)	73 (3 y)	68 (3 y)	71 (Kidney)	69 (3 y)	73 (3 y)
Cole et al 1994	Randomized	83 (Kidney)	69 (1 y)	81 (1 y)	83 (Kidney)	43 (1 y)[a]	78 (1 y)
Frey et al 1992	Randomized	67 (Kidney)	44 (NR)	87 (1 y)	71 (Kidney)	45 (NR)	84 (1 y)
Grino et al 1992[b]	Randomized	17 (Kidney/Pancreas)	88 (NR)	83 (2 y)	18 (Kidney/Pancreas)	88 (NR)	80 (2 y)
Hanto et al 1994	Randomized	72 (Kidney)	19 (3 m)	85 (3 y)	68 (Kidney)	15 (3 m)	82 (3 y)
Knechtle et al 1991	Sequential	59 (Kidney)	51 (3 y)	79 (3 y)	58 (Kidney)	37 (3 y)	78 (3 y)
Lefrancois et al 1990	Randomized	58 (Kidney/Pancreas)	40 (NR)	91 (1 y) Kidney	42 (Kidney)	45 (NR)	88 (1 y) Kidney
Light et al 1991	Concurrent[d]	15 (Kidney/Pancreas)	80 (11 ± 1.2 m)[c]	80 (1 y) Kidney	15 (Kidney/Pancreas)	67 (11.4 ± 1.2 m)[c]	93 (1 y) Kidney
		124 (Kidney)	40 (1 y)	81 (1 y) 78 (3 y)	116 (Kidney)	40 (1 y)	92 (1 y) 83 (3 y)
Lloveras et al 1992[a]	NR	45 (Kidney)	22 (6 m)	93 (1 y)	60 (Kidney)	32 (6 m)	89 (1 y)
Melzer et al 1990	NR	28 (Kidney/Pancreas)	NR [1.5 Kidney Rejection Episodes/Patient]	84 (1 y) Kidney	19 (Kidney/Pancreas)	NR [2.7 Kidney Rejection Episodes/Patient]	90 (1 y) Kidney
Steinmuller et al 1991	Randomized	25 (Kidney)	44 (NR)	88 (1 m) 84 (6 m)	26 (Kidney)	27 (NR)	84 (1 m) 84 (6 m)

NR = not reported; m = month; y = year
[a] p < 0.001
[b] Patients in this study did not receive azathioprine
[c] Mean ± standard deviation

OKT3 versus polyclonal antilymphocyte antibodies

A number of investigators have compared the use of OKT3 with polyclonal antilymphocyte globulin preparations for induction therapy[58-68] (Table 4.4). Initial therapy usually consisted in azathioprine and corticosteroids in addition to OKT3 or polyclonal antilymphocyte antibodies. In the majority of studies, length of treatment was the same with the monoclonal and polyclonal preparations. Cyclosporine administration was often delayed until creatinine determinations showed a decrease to a specified level. Overall study results demonstrate that induction of immunosuppression with OKT3 and polyclonal antilymphocyte antibodies is associated with similar percentages of patients undergoing rejection and graft survival.

What is the optimal regimen for OKT3 induction?

Dose of OKT3

Recently, OKT3 doses lower than the standard 5 mg/d have been evaluated in the hope of reducing the side effects and costs while maintaining efficacy. Both depletion and modulation of circulating CD3+ cells were observed with low OKT3 doses (1 to 2 mg/d), although modulation of CD3 was slower and reappearance of CD3+ cells in the circulation more rapid than with the standard 5 mg/day dose.[69-70] The main difference, however, between standard 5 mg/day and reduced doses is that OKT3 serum levels are considerably lower in the latter group.[70-71] This might be of importance, as it is unknown whether the full immunosuppressive effect of OKT3 is already achieved with depletion and modulation of CD3+ cells, allowing for reduced OKT3 doses, or whether it necessitates additional blockade of residual CD3 molecules, thereby requiring higher OKT3 doses to achieve sufficient serum levels. The limited experience with low OKT3 doses for induction therapy (Table 4.5) suggests that 2 mg OKT3/day could be as valuable as 5 mg/d.[70,73-76] This should clearly be further investigated in prospective, randomized trials that also include the high-risk recipients that benefited most from OKT3 prophylaxis.[57] Finally, it must be kept in mind that OKT3 dose requirements might differ for rejection and induction therapy, as well as between low- and high-risk recipients.

Table 4.5. Studies comparing different doses of OKT3 for induction therapy in renal transplantation

Study	Type of study	OKT3 regimen		Duration (days)	N° of patients	% patients with rejection episodes (follow-up)	% graft survival (follow-up)
		Patients	Dose (total, mg)				
Norman et al 1991	Consecutive	First graft	Standard (67)	14	29	38 (3 m)	90 (1 y)
			Low (22)	10	65	30 (3 m)	90 (1 y)
			Very low (9)	5	54	43 (3 m)	81 (1 y)
Schweizer et al 1992	Retrospective	High-risk	Standard (52)	10-14	10	NR[a]	70 (1 y)
			Low (35)	10-14	25	NR	96 (1 y)
Alloway et al 1992	Retrospective	Unselected	Standard (48)	7-10	27	52 (6 m)	10 (6 m)
			Low (23)	7-10	25	44 (6 m)	92 (6 m)
Alloway et al 1993	Prospective Randomized	First graft Low (23)	Standard (52)	7-14	25	0.72[b] (6 m)	96 (3 m)
				7-14	25	0.96 (6 m)	92 (3 m)
Norman et al 1994	Prospective Randomized	First graft	Standard (60)	12	13	0 (3 m)	92 (12 m)
			Low (24)	12	13	15 (3 m)	100 (12 m)

a: Not reported
b: Mean number of rejection per patient

Duration of OKT3 therapy

There is at present no study dealing with the optimal duration of OKT3 induction therapy in renal transplantation, but this issue has been addressed in cardiac transplant recipients.[77] Sixty-eight patients were consecutively allocated to receive OKT3 (5 mg/day) for either 10 (N = 34) or 14 (N = 34) days, together with steroids, azathioprine, and introduction of cyclosporinee on day 4. The 14-day course allowed for a reduced number of patients with rejection at 6 months as well as a higher percentage of patients withdrawn from maintenance steroids. These preliminary data suggest that 14-day OKT3 induction is superior to shorter therapy, although this should be confirmed in kidney transplant recipients.

Comparison of OKT3 for induction and first-line treatment

In order to refine treatment protocols for induction and treatment of rejection and to determine when it is best to intervene with OKT3, one group of investigators has directly compared the safety and efficacy of OKT3 for induction to its use for first-line treatment of rejection episodes.[78] In this prospective randomized trial, a significantly higher frequency of first-month rejections was observed in the group of 27 patients who received maintenance therapy with low-dose steroids and azathioprine and whose rejection episodes were treated for 10 days with first-line OKT3 (P < 0.001). The group with the lower rejection rate consisted of 28 patients who received OKT3 induction therapy for 30 days along with maintenance therapy of low-dose steroids and azathioprine (and high-dose steroids or antilymphocyte globulins for rejection). The 18-month graft survival was higher in the patients receiving OKT3 for induction than in patients receiving OKT3 for first-line treatment of rejection (89% vs 67%, respectively). This small study provides preliminary evidence that the benefits of OKT3 use for induction therapy may exceed those associated with its use at the time of rejection. However, the study results might have been improved in the group receiving OKT3 for first-line treatment of rejection if cyclosporine had been included in maintenance therapy.

OKT3 AND CYCLOSPORINE A: SYNERGY OR ANTAGONISM?

Whether the addition of cyclosporine A at the initiation of OKT3 therapy improves or antagonizes the efficacy of OKT3 therapy remains a matter of debate. On theoretical grounds, CsA could either add up to the immunosuppressive effects of OKT3 MoAb, or antagonize them by inhibiting the T-cell activation processes believed to be instrumental in immunosuppression. One retrospective study showed that maintenance of cyclosporine during OKT3 treatment of primary or rescue acute renal allograft rejection resulted in lower reversal rates and graft survival than its withdrawal (N° rejections reversed/total: 111/154 [72%] without CsA vs 42/74 [57%] with CsA, p = 0.025).[79] Along this line, data of the Collaborative Transplant Study registry showed that OKT3 prophylaxis improved 1-year kidney graft survival in high-risk recipients only if CsA administration was delayed (Dr. G. Opelz, ESOT Congress, Rhodos, October 1993). In addition to possible immunological antagonism between OKT3 and CsA, these negative results might also be due to their cumulative nephrotoxicity. On the opposite, Hricik et al observed no detrimental effect of CsA maintenance in a randomized, prospective study of OKT3 use for rescue therapy (actuarial graft survival at 1 year: 74% with CsA vs 69% without CsA).[43] Furthermore, the incidence of anti-OKT3 immunization was reduced in patients maintained on CsA during OKT3 treatment (3/27 vs 10/24, p < 0.02). Of interest, only low-dose CsA was administered in this study. Thus, the possibility that reduced CsA doses do not impair OKT3 efficacy and efficiently prevent anti-OKT3 antibody production should be further evaluated.

ADVERSE EVENTS ASSOCIATED WITH OKT3 ADMINISTRATION

Cytokine release syndrome

All patients experience to some extent the cytokine release syndrome after the initial OKT3 injection.[80] The most common symptoms are fever, chills, headaches, myalgia, nausea, vomiting and diarrhea.[5,13,38] Even though intense in some patients, these manifestations do not recur after the two or three initial OKT3 doses. Rarely, more serious complications such as pulmonary edema, encephalopathy, aseptic meningitis, convulsions or thrombosis of graft vessels (see below) may occur. The ability of OKT3 to induce multivalent cross-linking of both the T-cell receptor/CD3 complex and the monocyte Fc receptor results in T cell and monocyte activation.[81] This is accompanied by the release of several proinflammatory cytokines including tumor necrosis alpha (TNF-α), interferon gamma (IFN-γ), interleukin-2 and interleukin-6 into the circulation within hours after the initial OKT3 injection.[82-86] Recent studies, investigating cytokine gene expression in purified cell populations obtained from spleens of mice injected with an activating anti-CD3 antibody, indicate that T cells are the main source of TNF-α in this setting. Monocytes are also activated, as shown by their production of IL1 and IL6.[87] The toxicity of OKT3 is due to the synergy between TNF-α and IFN-α, as can also be observed after injection of both endotoxin and Staphylococcal enterotoxin B in mice. Indeed, MoAbs directed against either TNF-α[88-89] or IFN-γ[90] can prevent hypothermia, hypomotility, diarrhea, piloerection and even death induced by the activating 145-2C11 anti-CD3 MoAb in mice.

In addition to cytokines, OKT3 activates the complement system via the classical pathway as shown by increased levels of C3a and C4 metabolites within minutes of OKT3 injection.[17] Complement activation could synergise with cytokine and in particular could trigger early respiratory manifestations.[91] However, the occurrence of full-blown anti-CD3-induced toxicity in complement-deficient mice[34] as well as the lack of toxicity of a complement-binding non-mitogenic anti-T-cell receptor IgM MoAb[92] argues against a major role for complement activation in the pathogenesis of OKT3-associated toxicity.

In mouse and man, several strategies have been evaluated to attenuate the toxicity of activating anti-CD3 antibodies. These are aimed at reducing cytokine production, neutralizing the cytokines produced, or decreasing the production of secondary toxic mediators.

Drugs that reduce cytokine production

In mice, glucocorticosteroids if given in sufficient doses (> 30 mg/kg) and with the right timing (less than 4 h before anti-CD3 injection) almost completely suppress cytokine production and toxicity of anti-CD3 antibodies.[93] In man, glucorticosteroids are presently the only commercially available drug with clear efficiency in this setting. The optimal dose seems to be about 8 mg/kg of methylprednisolone (mPDS), given 1 to 4 h before OKT3 injection.[94] Larger doses of mPDS (30 mg/kg) did not result in lower TNF levels or better control of side effects.[95] Furthermore, these high doses of mPDS potentiate the procoagulant effects of OKT3 and might favor the occurrence of intragraft thromboses (see below).

Pentoxifylline (PTX), a drug that inhibits the enzyme phosphodiesterase, very efficiently diminishes anti-CD3-induced cytokine production, both in mice in vivo[96] as well as in man after stimulation of peripheral blood mononuclear cells with OKT3 in vitro.[97-98] However, the efficiency of PTX in man in vivo remains a matter of dispute. Leimenstoll observed that iv infusion of 500 mg PTX just prior to OKT3 injection in patients with renal graft rejection almost completely prevented TNF release,[99] a finding that we could not reproduce when PTX was given according to the same schedule but in renal transplant patients receiving OKT3 prophylactically.[100] Similarly, oral PTX attenuated the clinical manifestations of the cytokine release syndrome when OKT3 was used to treat steroid-resistant renal allograft rejection.[101] On the contrary, PTX did not influence either clinical manifestations or TNF and IL-6 levels when induction with OKT3 was given for kidney transplantation, despite achievement of adequate plasma levels of the drug and its active metabolites.[102] This suggests that PTX might display reduced activity in uremic patients. Further studies are needed to establish its efficiency in this situation.

Calcium-channel blockers, which in high doses block cytokine production in vitro, have also been administered to patients receiving OKT3 without any detectable effect.[103] These negative findings are probably due to the low doses used in vivo as compared to the concentrations achieved in in vitro experiments.

Interleukin-10, a cytokine with potent anti-inflammatory properties, might also attenuate OKT3 toxicity.[104] Indeed, IL-10 powerfully reduces TNF-α and IFN-γ production triggered by OKT3 by human PBMC in vitro.[98] In addition, recent in vivo studies in mice showed that injection of IL-10 efficiently inhibited TNF-α and IFN-γ production as well as clinical toxicity of anti-CD3 antibodies.[105] This together with a possible immunosuppressive effect of IL-10 on alloreactivity[106] could stimulate trials with recombinant human IL-10 in man.

Neutralization of cytokine

Neutralization of either TNF-α or IFN-γ was effective in attenuating anti-CD3 toxicity in mice. Similarly, anti-human TNF-α MoAb injected prior to the first dose of OKT3 markedly attenuated signs and symptoms in a clinical trial.[107]

Production of secondary mediators

Some of the side effects of proinflammatory cytokines like TNF-αTNF are mediated by second mediators among which are eicosanoids. The nonsteroidal antiinflammatory drug indomethacin (50 mg orally one hr prior to OKT3 followed by 25 mg every 6 hr for 2 days) reduced the incidence of fever, chills, arthralgias, and other constitutional symptoms after the first OKT3 injection, although there were no changes in TNF-α, IFN-γ or IL-2 serum levels.[108-109] However, the protection afforded by indomethacin was only moderate and its known nephrotoxicity together with the possible exacerbation of OKT3 encephalopathy[110] restricts its use in this context.

Thus, most of the above-mentioned drugs are either experimental (anti-TNF-α antibodies, IL-10) or have unproven efficacy (PTX, indomethacin, calcium-channel blockers). On practical grounds, the present recommendation to deal with the cytokine release syndrome is to administer 8 mg/kg mPDS 1 to 4 hours before the first OKT3 injection,[94] and to use antipyretic, antiemetic and antihistaminic drugs according to patient condition. In addition, the use of OKT3 as prophylaxis allows for the first injection to be given when the patient is anesthesized. By evaluating the intensity of side effects by a clinical score, we found that OKT3 first-dose reactions were considerably attenuated when administration during narcosis was compared to administration on the first post-operative day.[95]

OKT3 nephrotoxicity: from acute tubular necrosis to intragraft thrombosis

Part of the rationale for the prophylactic use of OKT3 in cadaver kidney transplantation was to delay cyclosporine therapy in the hope of reducing the incidence of post-operative acute tubular necrosis. However, the incidence of this complication has not been reduced by OKT3 use.[12,53] Furthermore, we made the unexpected observation that patients receiving OKT3 display an increased rate of post-operative dialysis requirement as compared to those treated with cyclosporine.[111] At that time, we administered only low doses of steroids as compared to other groups which did not observe this paradoxical effect of OKT3 (1 mg/kg mPDS before the first OKT3 injection, vs 4-8 mg/kg in the other centers). Later, we confirmed the critical role of steroid pretreatment, as increasing mPDS dose to 8 mg/kg before the first OKT3 injection allowed us to reduce dialysis requirement to the level encountered in our control recipients receiving cyclosporine.[112] This effect of steroids was probably due to reduced cytokine release with the increased dose.

Transient renal dysfunction has also been observed at the initiation of OKT3 anti-rejection therapy. Simpson et al observed signs of tubular toxicity in the urine sediment and a sharp increase in serum creatinine during the first 3 days of OKT3 therapy.[113] In a retrospective study, we extended these data by comparing evolution of kidney function during graft rejection treated with either OKT3 or mPDS.[114] The early increase in serum creatinine was significantly higher in OKT3 vs mPDS-treated patients. As in the prophylactic treatment, OKT3 nephrotoxicity appeared reversible and did not jeopardize the long-term graft outcome.

Several evidences now indicate that the renal dysfunction that may follow anti-CD3/TCR MoAbs use is related to the cytokine release they induce.[115] Indeed, injections in rodent and man of recombinant IL2, IFN-γ or TNF-α have been consistently reported to induce renal dysfunction, sometimes in association with acute tubular necrosis. Along this line, T10B9, an anti-TCR MoAb which leads to only minor increases in IFN-γ and TNF-α serum levels, does not induce nephrotoxicity.[92]

The observation that OKT3 possesses procoagulant properties which can precipitate intragraft thromboses and lead to transplant loss is a concern.[116] This adverse effect is related to the ability of OKT3 to activate the coagulation system as indicated by increased plasma levels of prothrombin fragments 1 + 2 (F 1 + 2) after the first OKT3 dose.[116-117] In vitro studies showed that OKT3 induces a procoagulant activity of the tissue-factor type on both endothelial cells and monocytes.[117-119] Even though all patients display transient systemic activation of the coagulation system after the first OKT3 dose, only a small number develop intragraft thrombosis. A multivariate analysis of the patients who received OKT3 at our institution revealed that pretreatment with high (30 mg/kg) rather than with ≤ 8 mg/kg m-PDS dose before the first OKT3 injection was associated with an increased incidence of thrombotic events (6 in 42 patients [14%] vs 7 in 189 patients [3.7%] who received ≤ 8 mg/kg m-PDS, p = 0.016).[119] The ability of glucocorticoids to synergize with OKT3 in the induction of tissue factor on monocytes might be the biological basis for this clinical observation.[119]

Our present strategy to prevent OKT3 nephrotoxicity is summarized in Table 4.6. Since these preventive measures were implemented, the incidence of post-operative dialysis fell from 106/198 (54%) in historical controls to 39/145 (27%) (p < 0.0001), and the incidence of early intragraft thromboses fell from 13/211 (6.2%) to 2/147 (1.4%) (p = 0.031). Thus, appropriate clinical management can efficiently prevent OKT3 nephrotoxicity.

Does OKT3 increases the risk of lymphoma?

During the first post-transplant year, the incidence of non-Hodgkin lymphoma in renal transplant recipients is about 0.5%.[120] This is at least 20 times more than in the general population. Indeed, heavy immunosuppression may lead to proliferation of EBV-infected B cells that have escaped T-cell control. There has been much concern in the transplant community because one group reported a dramatic increase in the incidence (11%) of early lymphomas in cardiac recipients immunosuppressed with OKT3.[121] A critical analysis of these data revealed that the development of lymphomas in this series was due to the administration of multiple courses of OKT3 therapy over a short period of time.[122] Multiple OKT3 courses obviously implies longer duration of profound immunosuppression, but also repetitive release of B-cell tropic cytokines at the initiation of each OKT3 course.[86] These mediators could synergize with the Epstein-Barr virus in the induction of pathological B cell proliferation. Although use of anti-lymphocyte agents–both ATG and OKT3–might increase lymphoma occurrence, the incidence as compared to patients who do not receive antibodies is increased by less than 0.5% (no ATG/OKT3 induction therapy, 50 lymphomas per 33.085 patients (0.15%); ATG, 43 lymphomas/10.660 patients (0.4%, p < 0.0001 vs no ATG/OKT3); OKT3, 8 lymphomas/1.396 patients (0.58%; p < 0.0001 vs no ATG/OKT3).[120] The impact of this figure on patient survival is not known, but is likely to be largely undetectable. Current opinion is that cumulative immunosuppression rather than use of any single agent is the critical factor affecting the rate of post-transplant lymphomas.

Table 4.6. Strategies for prevention of OKT3 nephrotoxicity

---

1. Avoid prophylactic OKT3 therapy in patients at risk for thrombosis:
   a. Patients with lupus anticoagulant or hemolytic-uremic syndrome
      as primary disease
   b. Recipients of kidneys from pediatric donors or adult donors with
      significant vascular lesions
2. Administer 8 mg/kg steroid pretreatment before the first OKT3 dose
3. Avoid hypovolemia
4. Administer a calcium channel blocker for the prevention of post-operative
   acute tubular necrosis
5. Give aspirin (100 mg/d) on the first post-operative day

Infections after OKT3 use

When prophylaxis with OKT3 was compared to cyclosporine A, data from the randomized Belgian study showed that the total number of infections was higher in OKT3 patients (124/1455 patient-months of risk exposure vs. 68/1320 in cyclosporine patients, p = 0.0006).[52] While most of this increase was due to urinary tract infections and to other benign infectious epiSodes, CMV disease also appeared more frequent in OKT3 patients (11/1455 episodes per patient-months of risk exposure vs. 3/1320 in cyclosporine patients, p = 0.06). In the USA randomized trial, the overall incidence of infections was similar in the OKT3 and cyclosporine treatment groups; however, the incidence of herpes simplex was 31% vs 19%, respectively (P = 0.060), and the incidence of CMV infection was 19% vs 5%, respectively (P = 0.055).[53] In a nonrandomized trial, 5 of 34 patients who received OKT3 developed CMV compared to 0 of 40 patients receiving early cyclosporine.[50] Thus, increased incidence of infections, including cytomegalovirus, was observed in patients receiving OKT3 induction. Most importantly, however, this had no impact on patient survival.[50,52,123,57] Improvements in the prevention and treatment of CMV disease by acyclovir or gancyclovir might help to reduce the incidence of this infection after OKT3 therapy.

As might be expected, the percentages of infections were similar when OKT3 therapy was compared to polyclonal anti-lymphocyte antibody treatment.[12] This probably reflects the similar immunosuppressive potency of these agents.

Anti-OKT3 antibody formation

This issue has been recently reviewed in detail by Dr. Chatenoud.[124-125] As OKT3 is a foreign protein, it can induce an antibody response against itself. Serum sickness has never been reported after OKT3 therapy, but anti-OKT3 antibodies may neutralize the injected OKT3 and result in therapeutic inefficiency. While this has been mainly observed during a second course of OKT3 administration, 10 to 15% of patients may develop neutralizing anti-OKT3 antibodies at the end of a first OKT3 course of 2 weeks duration.[126] Previous work has established that anti-OKT3 antibodies are likely to be neutralizing if they are: 1) produced in high titers ($\geq$ 1/1000 titer); 2) of the IgG isotype; 3) directed against idiotypic determinants of OKT3.[124] Patients appear to develop antibodies to OKT3 at varying frequencies. This may be due in part to lack of standardization of these assays. Indeed, widely discrepant results were reported when the same sera were assayed in different laboratories.[127]

Is it possible to efficiently retreat patients who got a previous course of OKT3 therapy? The answer is yes if the peak anti-OKT3 antibody titers observed after the first OKT3 course is $\leq$ 1:100. While the conventional ELISA used in these studies does not distinguish between blocking antiidiotypic and nonblocking antiisotypic anti-OKT3 antibodies, recent studies indicate that patients who harbor high titers of anti-OKT3 antibodies can be successfully retreated with OKT3 provided that blocking antibodies are absent.[128]

Presently, most centers administer azathioprine and corticosteroids together with OKT3 to prevent sensitization. With this protocol, about one-third of patients develop antiidiotypic antibodies, a figure that could be reduced to 10-15% with the addition of cyclosporine A.[129] It is likely that in the future, the use of humanized anti-CD3 antibodies will markedly reduce sensitization as has already been observed for other humanized antibodies.[124]

CONCLUSIONS

OKT3 is the first monoclonal antibody licensed for administration in humans. Widespread experience with OKT3 allowed to define several mechanisms by which it achieves immunosuppression in vivo, such as depletion, modulation and blocking of T-cell functions. The ability of one single MoAb to produce these multiple immunosuppressive effects probably accounts for its efficacy. In addition, several potential side effects of anti-lymphocyte antibody therapy such as sensitization and the release of cytokines have been described, and possible strategies to prevent them have been defined. Obviously, OKT3 is a MoAb of the first generation. The forthcoming antibodies will be humanized, thereby reducing sensitization, while the cytokine release syndrome can already be largely prevented with anti-CD3/TCR MoAbs unable to bind monocyte Fc receptors. One of the main challenge will be the clinical evaluation of the newer antibodies. Indeed, with 1-year graft survival now reaching more than 85%, carefully planned studies including sufficient number of patients will be required to demonstrate significant and medically relevant improvements of graft survival by new antibodies.

REFERENCES

1. Kung P, Goldstein G, Reinherz E, Schlossman S. Monoclonal antibodies defining distinctive human T cell surface antigens. Science 1979; 206:347-349.
2. Acuto O, Reinherz EL. The human T-cell receptor. Structure and function. N Engl J Med 1985; 312:1100-11.
3. Chang TW, Kung PC, Gingras SP, Goldstein G. Does OKT3 reacts with an antigen-recognition structure on human T cells? Proc Natl Acad Sci USA 1981; 78: 1805-1808.
4. Platsoucas CD, Good RA. Inhibition of cell-mediated cytotoxicity by monoclonal antibodies to human T cell antigens. Proc Natl Acad Sci USA 1981; 78:4500-4504.
5. Cosimi AB, Burton RC, Colvin RB, Goldstein G, Delmonico FL, LaQuaglia MP, Tolkoff-Rubin N, Rubin RH, Herrin JT, Russell PS. Treatment of acute renal allograft rejection with OKT3 monoclonal antibody. Transplantation 1981; 32:535-539.
6. Kreis H, Legendre C, Chatenoud L. OKT3 in organ transplantation. Transplant Rev 1991; 5:181-199.
7. Parlevliet KJ, Schellekens PT. Monoclonal antibodies in renal transplantation: a review. Transpl Int 1992; 5:234-46.
8. DeMattos A, Norman DJ. OKT3 for treatment of rejection in renal transplantation. Clin Transpl 1993; 7.
9. Peters H. The use of OKT3 in recipients of pancreatic, pulmonary, and bone marrow allografts. Clin Transplant 1993; 7:414-421.
10. Hockerstedt K. Treatment and prevention of liver allograft rejection with OKT3. Clin Transplant 1993; 7:403-413.
11. Renlund D. OKT3 for induction of immunosuppression and treatment of rejection in cardiac allograft recipients. Clin transplant 1993; 7:393-402.

12. Abramowicz D, Goldman M. OKT3 for induction of immunosuppression in renal transplantation. Clin Transpl 1993; 7:382-392.
13. Cosimi AB, Colvin RB, Burton RC, Rubin RH, Goldstein G, Kung PC, Hansen WP, Delmonico FL, Russell PS. Use of monoclonal antibodies to T-cell subsets for immunologic monitoring and treatment in recipients of renal allografts. N Engl J Med 1981; 305:308-314.
14. Chatenoud L, Baudrihaye JM, Kreis H, Bach JF. Human in vivo antigenic modulation induced by the anti-T cell OKT3 monoclonal antibody. Eur J Immunol 1982; 12:979-982.
15. Dustin M, Springer T. T-cell receptor cross-linking transiently stimulates adhesiveness through LFA-1. Nature 1989; 341:619-624.
16. Bergese SD, Pelletier RP, Ohye RG, Vallera DA, Orosz CG. Treatment of mice with anti-CD3 mAb induces endothelial vascular cell adhesion molecule-1 expression. Transplantation 1994; 57:711-7.
17. Raasveld MH, Bemelman FJ, Schellekens PT, van DF, van DA, van RE, Hack CE, ten BI. Complement activation during OKT3 treatment:a possible explanation for respiratory side effects. Kidney Int 1993; 43:1140-9.
18. Russell JH, Rush BJ, Abrams SI, Wang R. Sensitivity of T cells to anti-CD3-stimulated suicide is independent of functional phenotype. Eur J Immunol 1992; 22:1655-8.
19. Wong J, Eylath A, Ghobrial I, Colvin R. The mechanisms of anti-CD3 monoclonal antibodies: mediation of cytolysis by inter-T cell bridging. Transplantation 1990; 50:683-689.
20. Tsoukas C, Fox R, Slovin S et al. Molecular interactions in human T-cell mediated cytotoxicity to EBV. I. Blocking of effector cell function by monoclonal antibody OKT3. Cell Immunol 1982; 69:113-119.
21. Landegren U, Ramstedt U, Axberg I, Ullberg M, Jondal M, Wigzell H. Selective inhibition of human T cell cytotoxicity at levels of target recognition or initiation of lysis by monoclonal OKT3 and Leu-2a antibodies. J Exp Med 1982; 155:1579-1584.
22. Tsoukas C, Carson D, Fong S, Vaughan J. Molecular interactions in human T-cell mediated cytotoxixity to EBV. II. Monoclonal antibody OKT3 inhibits a post-killer-target recognition/adhesion step. J Immunol 1982; 129:1421-1425.
23. Nau GJ, Moldwin RL, Lancki DW, Kim DK, Fitch FW. Inhibition of IL 2-driven proliferation of murine T lymphocyte clones by supraoptimal levels of immobilized anti-T cell receptor monoclonal antibody. J Immunol 1987; 139:114-122.
24. Webb S, Sprent J. Downregulation of T cell responses by antibodies to the T cell receptor. J Exp Med 1987; 165:584-589.
25. Williams ME, Lichtman AH, Abbas AK. Anti-CD3 antibody induces unresponsiveness to IL-2 in Th1 clones but not in Th2 clones. J Immunol 1990; 144:1208-1214.
26. Jenkins MK, Chen C, Jung G, Mueller DL, Schwartz RH. Inhibi-

tion of antigen-specific proliferation of type 1 murine T cell clones after stimulation with immobilized anti-CD3 monoclonal antibody. J Immunol 1990; 144:16-22.

27. Schwartz R. A cell culture model for T lymphocyte clonal anergy. Science 1990; 248:1349-1356.

28. Davis LS, Wacholtz MC, Lipsky PE. The induction of T cell unresponsiveness by rapidly modulating CD3. J Immunol 1989; 142:1084-1094.

29. Pantaleo G, Olive D, Poggi A, Pozzan T, Moretta L, Moretta A. Antibody-induced modulation of the CD3/T cell receptor complex causes T cell refractoriness by inhibiting the early metabolic steps involved in T cell activation. J Exp Med 1987; 166.

30. Dubois PM, Andris F, Shapiro RA, L.K. G, Kaufman M, Urbain J, Ledbetter JA, Leo O. T cell long-term hyporesponsiveness follows antigen receptor engagement and results from defective signal transduction. Eur J Immunol 1994; 24.

31. Williams ME, Shea CM, Lichtman AH, Abbas AK. Antigen receptor-mediated anergy in resting T lymphocytes and T cell clones. J Immunol 1992; 149:1921-1926.

32. Wolf H, Müller Y, Salmen S, Wilmanns W, G. J. Induction of anergy in resting human T lymphocytes by immobilized anti-CD3 antibodies. Eur J Immunol 1994; 24:1410-1417.

33. Anasetti C, Tan P, Hansen JA, Martin PJ. Induction of specific nonresponsiveness in unprimed human T cells by anti-CD3 antibody and alloantigen. J Exp Med 1990; 172:1691-1700.

34. Mackie JD, Pankewycz OG, Bastos MG, Kelley VE, Strom TB. Dose-related mechanisms of immunosuppression mediated by murine anti-CD3 monoclonal antibody in pancreatic islet cell transplantation and delayed-type hypersensitivity. Transplantation 1990; 49:1150-1154.

35. Nicolls MR, Aversa GG, Pearce NW, Spinelli A, Berger MF, Gurley KE, Hall BM. Induction of long-term specific tolerance to allografts in rats by therapy with an anti-CD3-like monoclonal antibody. Transplantation 1993; 55:459-68.

36. Heidecke CD, Hancock WW, Jakobs F, Westerholt S, Sewzcik T, Deusch K, Zanti N, Kurrle R, Kupiec-Weglinski J. TCRa/b targeted therapy in the rat: pretreatment with R73 monoclonal antibody induces profound immunological anergy and long-term allograft survival. Transplant Proc 1993; 25:540-542.

37. Knight RJ, Kurrle R, Stepkowski S, Serino F, Chou TC, Kahan BD. Synergistic immunosuppressive actions of cyclosporine with a mouse anti-rat a/b-T cell receptor monoclonal antibody. Transplantation 1994; 57:1544-1548.

38. A randomized clinical trial of OKT3 monoclonal antibody for acute rejection of cadaveric renal transplants. Ortho Multicenter Transplant Study Group. N Engl J Med 1985; 313:337-42.

39. Deierhoi MH, Barber WH, Curtis JJ, Julian BA, Luke RG, Hudson

S, Barger BO, Diethelm AG. A comparison of OKT3 monoclonal antibody and corticosteroids in the treatment of acute renal allograft rejection. Am J Kid Dis 1988; XI:86-89.

40. Tesi RJ, Elkhammas EA, Henry ML, Ferguson RM. OKT3 for primary therapy of the first rejection episode in kidney transplants. Transplantation 1993; 55:1023-9.

41. Suthanthiran M, Wiebe ME, Stenzel KH. Effect of immunosuppressants on OKT3 associated T cell activation:clinical implications. Kidney Int 1987; 32:362-367.

42. De Mattos AM, Norman DJ. OKT3 for treatment of rejection in renal transplantation. Clin Transplant 1993; 7:374-381.

43. Hricik D, Mayes J, Schulak J. Inhibition of anti-OKT3 antibody generation by cyclosporine-results of a prospective, randomized trial. Transplantation 1990; 50:237-240.

44. Hesse UJ, Wienand P, Baldamus C, Ams W. Preliminary results of a prospectively randomized trial of ALG Vs OKT3 for steroid-resistant rejection after renal transplantation in the early postoperative period. Transplant Proc 1990; 22:2273-2274.

45. Alamartine E, Bellakoul R, Berthoux F. Randomized prospective study comparing OKT3 and antithymocyte globulins for treatment of the first acute cellular rejection of kidney allografts. Transplant Proc 1994; 26:273-4.

46. Blümke M, Kirste G, Wanner U, Wilms H. Single center randomized trial using ATG v OKT3 treatment in steroid resistant rejection crises after kidney transplantation. Transplant Proc 1989; 21:1747.

47. Delaney VB, Campbell WG, Nasr SA, McCue PA, Warshaw B, Whelchel JD. Efficacy of OKT3 monoclonal antibody therapy in steroid-resistant, predominantly vascular acute rejection. Transplantation 1988; 45:743-748.

48. Schroeder TJ, Weiss MA, Smith RD, Stephens GW, M.R. F. The efficacy of OKT3 in vascular rejection. Transplantation 1991; 51:312-315.

49. Colon S, Pouteil-Noble C, Ecochard R, Lacavalerie B, Touraine J. Lésions histologiques pronostiquées de la perte du greffon lors du premier rejet. Etude cas-témoin. Néphrologie 1993; 14.

50. Benvenisty AI, Cohen D, Sregall MD, Hardy MA. Improved results using OKT3 as induction immunosuppression in renal allografts recipients with delayed graft function. Transplantation 1990; 49:321-327.

51. Dafoe D, Bromberg J, Grossman R, Tomaszewski J, Zmijewski C, Perloff L, Naji A, Asplund M, Alfrey E, Sack M, Zellers L, Kearns J, Barker C. Renal transplantation despite a positive antiglobulin crossmatch with and without prophylactic OKT3. Transplantation 1991; 51:762-768.

52. Abramowicz D, Goldman M, De Pauw L, Vanherweghem JL,

Kinnaert P, Vereerstraeten P. The long-term effects of prophylactic OKT3 monoclonal antibody in cadaver kidney transplantation—a single-center, prospective, randomized study. Transplantation 1992; 54:433-7.

53. Norman DJ, Kahana L, Stuart FJ, Thistlethwaite JJ, Shield CE, Monaco A, Dehlinger J, Wu SC, Van HA, Haverty TP. A randomized clinical trial of induction therapy with OKT3 in kidney transplantation. Transplantation 1993; 55:44-50.

54. Kahana L, Ackerman J, Lefor W et al. Use of Orthoclone OKT3 for prophylaxis of rejection and induction in initial nonfonction in kidney transplantation. Transplant Proc 1990; 22:1755-1758.

55. Schroeder T, First M, Mansour R, Alexander J, Penn I. Prophylactic use of OKT3 in immunologic high-risk cadaver renal transplant recipients. Am J Kid Dis 1989; 14:14-18.

56. Cecka JM, Gjertson D, Terasaki PI. Do prophylactic antilymphocyte globulins (ALG and OKT3) improve renal transplant survival in recipient and donor high-risk groups? Transplant Proc 1993; 25:548-549.

57. Abramowicz D, Norman D, Goldman M, De Pauw L, Kinnaert P, Kahana L, Thistlethwaite J, Shield C, Monaco A, Vanherweghem J, Vereerstraeten P. OKT3 prophylaxis improves long-term renal graft survival in high-risk patients as compared to cyclosporine A: combined results from the prospective, randomized Belgian and U.S. studies. Transplant Proc 1995; In press:

58. Lefrancois N, Raffaele P, Martinenghi S et al. Prophylactic polyclonal versus monoclonal antibodies in kidney and pancreas transplantation. Transpl Proc 1990; 22:632-633.

59. Melzer J, D'allessandro A, Kalayoglu M, Pirsch J, Belzer F, Sollinger H. The use of OKT3 in combined pancreas-kidney allotransplantation. Transplant Proc 1990; 22:634-635.

60. Steinmuller DR, Hayes JM, Novick AC, Streem SB, Hodge E, Slavis S, Martinez A, Graneto D, G. P. Comparison of OKT3 with ALG for prophylaxis for patients with acute renal failure after cadaveric renal transplantation. Transplantation 1991; 52:67-71.

61. Knechtle SJ, Pirsch JD, Groshek M, Reed A, D'Alessandro AM, Kalayoglu M, Belzer FO, Sollinger HW. OKT3 vs ALG induction therapy in combined pancreas-kidney transplantation. Transplant Proc 1991; 23:1581-1582.

62. Light JA, Jonsson J, Khawand N, Ali A, Aquino A, Currier CB, Romolo J, Gonzalez J, Korb S. Sequential Immunosuppression: Three years' experience in 240 cadaveric renal transplants. Transplant Proc 1991; 23:1032-1035.

63. Lloveras J, Puig JM, Oliveras A, Orfila A, Comerma I, Aubia J, Masramon J. Prophylaxis with a short course of OKT3 in renal transplantation: comparative analysis with recipients treated either with prophylactic ATG or with CyA. Transplant Proc 1992; 24:43-4.

64. Frey DJ, Matas AJ, Gillingham KJ, Canafax D, Payne WD, Dunn DL, Sutherland DER, Najarian JS. Sequential therapy—a prospective randomized trial of MALG versus OKT3 for prophylactic immunosuppression in cadaver renal allograft recipients. Transplantation 1992; 54:50-56.

65. Grino JM, Castelao AM, Seron D, Gonzalez C, Galceran JM, Gil VS, Andres E, Mestre M, Torras J, Alsina J. Antilymphocyte globulin versus OKT3 induction therapy in cadaveric kidney transplantation: a prospective randomized study. Am J Kidney Dis 1992; 20:603-10.

66. Broyer M, Gagnadoux MF, Guest G, Arsan A, Beurton D, Revillon Y, Niaudet P. Prophylactic OKT3 monoclonal antibody versus Antilymphocyte Globulins: a prospective, randomized study in 148 first cadaver kidney grafts. Transplant Proc 1993; 25:570-571.

67. Cole EH, Cattran DC, Farewell VT, Aprile M, Bear RA, Pei YP, Fenton SS, Tober JAL, Cardella CJ. A comparison of rabbit antithymocyte serum and OKT3 as prophylaxis against renal allograft rejection. Transplantation 1994; 57:60-67.

68. Hanto DW, Jendrisak MD, So SK, McCullough CS, Rush TM, Michalski SM, Phelan D, Mohanakumar T. Induction immunosuppression with antilymphocyte globulin or OKT3 in cadaver kidney transplantation. Results of a single institution prospective randomized trial. Transplantation 1994; 57:377-84.

69. Henell KR, Bakke A, Kenny TA, Kimball JA, Barry JM, Norman DJ. Degree of Modulation of cell-surface CD3 by anti-lymphocyte therapies. Transplant Proc 1991; 23:1070-1071.

70. Norman D, Kimball J, Benett W, Shihab F, Batiuk T, Meyer M, Barry J. A prospective, double-blind, randomized study of high-versus low-dose OKT3 induction immunosuppression in cadaveric renal transplantation. Transplant Int 1994; 7:356-361.

71. Parlevliet KJ, ten Berge RJM, Raasveld MHM, Surachno J, J.M.W, Schellekens PTA. Low-dose OKT3 induction therapy following renal transplantation: a controlled study. Nephrol Dial Transplant 1994; 9:698-703.

72. Alloway R, Kotb M, Hathaway D, Ohman M, Strain S, Gaber A. The pharmacokinetic profile of standard and low-dose OKT3 induction immunosuppression in renal transplant recipients. Transplantation 1994; 58:249-253.

73. Norman DJ, Barry JM, Benett WM, Munson JL, Meyer M, Henell K, Kimball J, Hubert B. OKT3 for induction immunosuppression in renal transplantation: a comparative study of high versus low doses. Transplant Proc 1991; 23:1052-1054.

74. Schweizer RT, Roper L, Hull D, Bartus SA. Low-dose OKT3 for cadaveric renal transplantation. Transplant Proc 1992; 24:2592-3.

75. Alloway RR, Kotb M, Gaber LW, Vera SR, Boskey F, Gaber AO. Standard versus low-dose OKT3 induction therapy of cadaveric renal transplants: comparison of outcome data versus OKT3 dose and

serum levels. Clin Transplant 1992; 46:468-472.

76. Alloway R, Kotb M, Hathaway DK, Gaber LW, Vera SR, Gaber AO. Randomized double-blind study of standard versus low-dose OKT3 induction therapy in renal allograft recipients. Am J Kidney Dis 1993; 22:36-43.

77. Hegewald M, O'Conell J, Renlund D et al. OKT3 monoclonal antibody given for ten versus fourteen days as immunosuppressive prophylaxis in heart transplantation. J Heart Transplant 1989; 8:303-310.

78. Kreis H, Chkoff N, Chatenoud L, Debure A, Lacombe M, Chretien Y, Legendre C, Caillat S, Bach JF. A randomized trial comparing the efficacy of OKT3 used to prevent or to treat rejection. Transplant Proc 1989; 21:1741-1744.

79. Hirsch RL, Layton PC, Barnes LA, Kremer AB, Goldstein G. Orthoclone OKT3 treatment of acute renal allograft rejection in patients receiving maintenance cyclosporine therapy. Transplant Proc 1987.

80. Kreis H. Adverse events associated with OKT3 immunosuppression in the prevention or treatment of allograft rejection. Clin Transplantation 1993; 7:431-446.

81. Van Wauwe J, De Mey J, Goossens J. OKT3:a monoclonal antibody with potent mitogenic properties. J Immunol 1980; 124:2708-2713.

82. Abramowicz D, Schandene L, Goldman M, Crusiaux A, Vereerstraeten P, De Pauw L, Wybran J, Kinnaert P, Dupont E, Toussaint C. Release of tumor necrosis factor, interleukin-2, and gamma-interferon in serum after injection of OKT3 monoclonal antibody in kidney transplant recipients. Transplantation 1989; 47:606-8.

83. Chatenoud L, Ferran C, Reuter A, Legendre C, Gevaert Y, Kreis H, Franchimont P, Bach JF. Systemic reaction to the anti-T-cell monoclonal antibody OKT3 in relation to serum levels of tumor necrosis factor and interferon-gamma. N Engl J Med 1989; 320:1420-1.

84. Bloemena E, ten Berge IJM, Surachno J, Wilmink JM. Kinetics of interleukin 6 during OKT3 treatment in renal allograft recipients. Transplantation 1990; 50:330-331.

85. Gaston RS, Deierhoi MH, Patterson T, Prasthofer E, Julian BA, Barber WH, Laskow DA, Diethelm AG, Curtis JJ. OKT3 first-dose reaction: association with T cell subsets and cytokine release. Kidney Int 1991; 39:141-148.

86. Goldman M, Gérard C, Abramowicz D, Schandené L, Durez P, De Pauw L, Kinnaert P, Vereerstraeten P, Velu T. Induction of interleukin-6 and interleukin-10 by the OKT3 monoclonal antibody: possible relevance to posttransplant lymphoproliferative disorders. Clin Transplant 1992; 6:265-268.

87. Ferran C, Dautry F, Merite S, Sheehan K, Schreiber R, Grau G, Bach JF, Chatenoud L. Anti-tumor necrosis factor modulates anti-CD3-triggered T cell cytokine gene expression in vivo. J Clin Invest 1994; 93:2189-96.

88. Alegre M, Vandenabeele P, Flamand V, Moser M, Leo O, Abramowicz D, Urbain J, Fiers W, Goldman M. Hypothermia and hypoglycemia induced by anti-CD3 monoclonal antibody in mice: role of tumor necrosis factor. Eur J Immunol 1990; 20:707-10.

89. Ferran C, Dy M, Sheehan K, Schreiber R, Grau G, Bluestone J, Bach JF, Chatenoud L. Cascade modulation by anti-tumor necrosis factor monoclonal antibody of interferon-gamma, interleukin 3 and interleukin 6 release after triggering of the CD3/T cell receptor activation pathway. Eur J Immunol 1991; 21:2349-53.

90. Matthys P, Dillen C, Proost P, Heremans H, Van DJ, Billiau A. Modification of the anti-CD3-induced cytokine release syndrome by anti-interferon-gamma or anti-interleukin-6 antibody treatment: protective effects and biphasic changes in blood cytokine levels. Eur J Immunol 1993; 23:2209-16.

91. Bûsing M, Mellert J, Greger B, Hopt U. Acute pulmonary insufficiency due to OKT3 therapy. Transplant Proc 1990; 22:1779.

92. Waid TH, Lucas BA, Thompson JS, Brown SA, Munch L, Prebeck RJ, Jezek D. Treatment of acute cellular rejection with T10B9.1A-31 or OKT3 in renal allograft recipients. Transplantation 1992; 53:80-6.

93. Alegre ML, Vandenabeele P, Depierreux M, Florquin S, Deschodt Lanckman M, Flamand V, Moser M, Leo O, Urbain J, Fiers W, Goldman M. Cytokine release syndrome induced by the 145-2C11 anti-CD3 monoclonal antibody in mice: prevention by high doses of methylprednisolone. J Immunol 1991; 146:1184-91.

94. Norman D, Chatenoud L, Cohen D, Goldman M, Shield C. Consensus statement regarding OKT3-induced cytokine-release syndrome and human antimouse antibodies. Transplant Proc 1993; 25:89-92.

95. Doutrelepont JM, Abramowicz D, Borre B, Lemoine A, De PL, Kinnaert P, Vereerstraeten P, Vanherweghem JL, Goldman M. Prophylactic OKT3: practical considerations for the prevention of first-dose reactions. Transplant Proc 1993;

96. Alegre ML, Gastaldello K, Abramowicz D, Kinnaert P, Vereerstraeten P, De PL, Vandenabeele P, Moser M, Leo O, Goldman M. Evidence that pentoxifylline reduces anti-CD3 monoclonal antibody-induced cytokine release syndrome. Transplantation 1991; 52:674-9.

97. Schandene L, Vandenbussche P, Crusiaux A, Alegre ML, Abramowicz D, Dupont E, Content J, Goldman M. Differential effects of pentoxifylline on the production of tumour necrosis factor-alpha (TNF-alpha) and interleukin-6 (IL-6) by monocytes and

T cells. Immunology 1992; 76:30-4.

98. Schandene L, Gerard C, Crusiaux A, Abramowicz D, Velu T, Goldman M. Interleukin-10 inhibits OKT3-induced cytokine release:in vitro comparison with pentoxifylline. Transplant Proc 1993; 25:55-56.

99. Leimenstoll G, Zabel P, Schroeder P, Schlaak M, Niedermayer W. Suppression of OKT3-induced tumor necrosis factor alpha formation by pentoxifylline in renal transplant recipients. Transplant Proc 1993; 25:561-563.

100. Abramowicz D, Pradier O, Schandene L, Crusiaux A, De Pauw L, Vanherweghem J, Capel P, Kinnaert P, Vereerstraeten P, Goldman M. Pentoxifylline prevents TNF production and activation of coagulation induced by OKT3 in vitro but not in vivo. J Am Soc Nephrol 1993; 4:921.

101. Vincenti FG, Vasconcelos M, Birnbaum JL, Tomlanovich SJ, Amend WJ, Melzer JS, Snyder JP. Pentoxifylline reduces the first-dose reactions following OKT3. Transplant Proc 1993; 25:57-59.

102. DeVault GJ, Kohan DE, Nelson EW, Holman JJ. The effects of oral pentoxifylline on the cytokine release syndrome during inductive OKT3. Transplantation 1994; 57:532-40.

103. Richard EA, Lorber MI, Marks WH, Bia MJ. Are calcium channel blockers protective against first-dose reactions to OKT3? Transplantation 1992; 54:372-4.

104. Howard M, Ogarra A, Ishida H, Malefyt RD, Devries J. Biological Properties of Interleukin-10. J Clin Immunol 1992; 12:239-247.

105. Donckier V, Flament V, Gerard C, Abramowicz D, Vandenabeele P, Wissing M, Delvaux A, Fiers W, Leo O, Velu T et al. Modulation of the release of cytokines and reduction of the shock syndrome induced by anti-CD3 monoclonal antibody in mice by interleukin-10. Transplantation 1994; 57:1436-9.

106. Delvaux A, Donckier V, Bruyns C, Florquin S, Gerard C, Amraoui Z, Abramowicz D, Goldman M, Velu T. Effects of systemic administration of rIL-10 in an in vivo model of alloreactivity. Transplantation 1994; In press:

107. Charpentier B, Hiesse C, Lantz O, Ferran C, Stephens S, O'Shaugnessy D, Bodmer M, Benoit G, Bach JF, Chatenoud L. Evidence that antihuman tumor necrosis factor monoclonal antibody prevents OKT3-induced acute syndrome. Transplantation 1992; 54:997-1002.

108. Shield C3, Kahana L, Pirsch J, Vergne MP, First MR, Schroeder TJ, Cohen D, Norman DJ, Monaco A, Martinez A et al. Use of indomethacin to minimize the adverse reactions associated with orthoclone OKT3 treatment of kidney allograft rejection. Transplantation 1992; 54:164-6.

109. First MR, Schroeder TJ, Hariharan S, Weiskittel P. Reduction of the initial febrile response to OKT3 with indomethacin. Trans-

plant Proc 1993.

110. Chan G, Weinstein S, Wright C, Bowers V, Alveranga D, Shires D, Ackerman J, Lefor W, Kahana L. Encephalopathy associated with OKT3 administration. Possible interactions with indomethacin. Transplantation 1991; 52:148-150.

111. Toussaint C, De Pauw L, Vereerstraeten P, Kinnaert P, Abramowicz D, Goldman M. Possible nephrotoxicity of the prophylactic use of OKT3 monoclonal antibody after cadaveric renal transplantation. Transplantation 1989; 48:524-6.

112. Goldman M, Abramowicz D, De Pauw L, Alegre ML, Widera I, Vereerstraeten P, Kinnaert P. OKT3-induced cytokine release attenuation by high-dose methylprednisolone [letter]. Lancet 1989; 2:802-3.

113. Simpson MA, Madras PN, Cornaby AJ, Etienne T, Dempsey RA, Clowes GH, Monaco AP. Sequential determinations of urinary cytology and plasma and urinary lymphokines in the management of renal allograft recipients. Transplantation 1989; 47:218-23.

114. Goldman M, Van LJ, Abramowicz D, De PL, Kinnaert P, Vereerstraeten P. Evolution of renal function during treatment of kidney graft rejection with OKT3 monoclonal antibody. Transplantation 1990; 50:158-9.

115. Omitted in proofs.

116. Abramowicz D, Pradier O, Marchant A, Florquin S, De Pauw L, Vereerstraeten P, Kinnaert P, Vanherweghem JL, Goldman M. Induction of thromboses within renal grafts by high-dose prophylactic OKT. Lancet 1992; 339:777-8.

117. Pradier O, Marchant A, Abramowicz D, De Pauw L, Vereerstraeten P, Kinnaert P, Vanherweghem JL, Capel P, Goldman M. Procoagulant effect of the OKT3 monoclonal antibody: involvement of tumor necrosis factor. Kidney Int 1992; 42:1124-9.

118. Pradier O, Abramowicz D, Capel P, Goldman M. Procoagulant properties of OKT3 at the monocyte level: inhibition by pentoxifylline. Transplant Proc 1993.

119. Abramowicz D, Pradier O, De Pauw L, Kinnaert P, Mat O, Surquin M, Doutrelepont J, Vanherweghem J, Capel P, Vereerstraeten P, Goldman M. High-dose glucocorticosteroids increase the procoagulant effects of OKT3. Kidney Int 1994; In press.

120. Opelz G, Henderson R. Incidence of non-Hodgkin lymphoma in kidney and heart transplant recipients. Lancet 1993; 342:1514-1516.

121. Swinnen L, Costanzo-Nordin M, Fisher S, O'Sullivan E, Johnson M, Heroux A, Dizikes G, Pifarre R, Fisher R. Increased incidence of lymphoproliferative disorder after immunosuppression with the monoclonal antibody OKT3 in cardiac-transplant recipients. N Engl J Med 1990; 323:1723-1728.

122. Abramowicz D, Goldman M, De Pauw L, Doutrelepont JM, Kinnaert P, Vanherweghem J, Vereerstraeten P. OKT3 and post-

transplantation lymphoproliferative disorders. N Eng J Med 1991; 324:1438-1439.

123. Norman DJ, Kahana L, Stuart F, Thistlethwaite RJ, Shield CF, Monaco A, Dehlinger J, Wu SC, Van Horn A, Haverty TP. A randomized clinical trial of induction therapy with OKT3 in kidney transplantation. Transplantation 1993; 55:44-50.

124. Chatenoud L. Humoral immune response against OKT3. Transplant Proc 1993; 25:68-73.

125. Chatenoud L. Immunologic monitoring during OKT3 therapy. Clin Transplant 1993; 7:422-430.

126. Abramowicz D, Goldman M, Mat O, Estermans G, Crusiaux A, Vanherweghem J, De Pauw L, Kinnaert P, P V. OKT3 serum levels as a guide for prophylactic therapy: a pilot study in kidney transplant recipients. Transplant Int 1994; 7:258-263.

127. Kimball JA, Norman DJ, Shield CF, Schroeder TJ, Lisi P, Garovoy M, O'Connell JB, Stuart F, McDiarmid SV, Wall W. OKT3 antibody response study (OARS): a multicenter comparative study. Transplant Proc 1993.

128. Legendre C, Kreis H, Bach JF, Chatenoud L. Prediction of successful allograft rejection retreatment with OKT3. Transplantation 1992; 53:87-90.

129. Chatenoud L, Bach JF. Therapeutic monoclonal antibodies in transplantation. Transplant Proc 1993; 25:473-474.

CHAPTER 5

MONOCLONAL ANTIBODIES TO ADHESION MOLECULES IN BONE MARROW AND ORGAN TRANSPLANTATION

Alain Fischer, M. Cavazzana-Calvo, N. Jabado and S. Sarnacki

A number of adhesion molecules have been characterized in the recent past. Molecules belonging to three families, i.e. selectins, integrins and members of the immunoglobulin superfamily mediate major events of immune reactions.[1,2] These events include migration of naïve cells to lymphoid organs (homing), adhesion of T cells to antigen-presenting cells, adhesion between effector helper or cytotoxic T cells and B cells or target cells respectively, migration of lymphocytes (as well as monocytes and granulocytes) from the blood stream to sites of immune reaction. T-cell activation and migration are obvious key phenomena in the process of graft rejection and graft versus host disease (GVHD). Adhesion molecules therefore represent logical targets for immunointervention aim at preventing graft rejection. In this chapter, we review the current experimental and clinical data on the in vivo use of anti-adhesion molecule antibodies in the field of transplantation.

Table 5.1 lists adhesion molecules involved in both T-cell activation and lymphocyte migration, i.e. interaction with endothelial cells. Resting T cells loosely interact with other cells mostly through low avidity state LFA-1/ICAMs and CD2/LFA-3 interactions.[3-6] Antigen recognition triggers a rapid transient and dramatic

Monoclonal Antibodies in Transplantation, edited by Lucienne Chatenoud. © 1995 R.G. Landes Company.

upregulation of the LFA-1-mediated adhesion pathway by increasing LFA-1 avidity (recruitment of LFA-1 molecules to areas of cell-to-cell contact), clustering, cytoskeletal association with cytoskeleton and enhanced affinity through conformational changes.[7,8] ICAM-3 binding to LFA-1 on antigen-presenting cells (such as dendritic cells), as well as CD2 or CD28 molecules, may also contribute to upregulate of LFA-1 avidity, these events likely converging to amplify and prolong adhesion between immunocompetent cells.[9,10] This limited period of high avidity adhesion creates optimal cell-to-cell interaction and thereby promotes intracellular signaling leading to lymphokine delivery or cell cytotoxicity.[11] In tissues, local ongoing immune response through release of cytokines such as IL-1, interferon γ and TNF leads within hours to the surface induction of ICAM-1 molecules expression by many cell types thus favoring interaction with activated T cells.[1,2]

Resting lymphocytes do not adhere to non-activated endothelial cells. Local activation (by infection or onset of an immune response) induces the expression of selectins such as E-selectin by endothelial cells as well as the activation of integrins LFA-1 and

Table 5.1. Main molecules involved in T/APC or target cell adhesion (A) and in lymphocyte/endothelial cell interaction (B)

A.	T	APC
		target cell
	CD2	LFA-3
	ICAM-3	LFA-1*
	LFA-1	ICAM-1 (2, 3*)

* expression restricted to leukocytes

B.	Lymphocyte	Endothelial cells
Rolling		
	L-selectin	Gly-Cam 1
		CD34
		Mad Cam 1
	CLA	E-selectin*
Adhesion		
	LFA-1	ICAM-2
		ICAM-1*
	VLA-4	VCAM-1*

* expression induced by local secretion of cytokines (IL-1, interferon γ, TNF)

VLA-4 on lymphocytes. In a first step, transient short-term interactions between selectins and sialyl lewis carbohydrates expressed by certain proteins, lymphocyte circulation flow in the blood stream, promoting cells rolling over endothelial cells. This subsequently facilitates sticking of leukocytes and transendothelial migration by successive adhesion steps using integrin/ligand molecular pathways (LFA-1 ICAM-1 and VLA-4: VCAM-1 interaction).[1,2]

THE LEUKOCYTE ADHESION DEFICIENCY (LAD)

LAD type I syndrome is a rare autosomal recessive disorder consisting of a defective membrane expression of the β2 leukocyte integrins, i.e., LFA-1, Mac-1, p150,95, on all leukocytes. Absence or abnormal β2 (CD18) expression results from heterogeneous mutations in the gene encoding for the shared β sub-unit, resulting in impaired synthesis or deficient association with the α chain leukocytes from LAD patients and are unable to adhere to endothelium and migrate into tissues causing patients to develop severe, persisting bacterial infections. Because the disease is life-threatening, HLA-identical allogeneic bone marrow transplantation (BMT) has been used as a curative therapy with success. Attempts at HLA partially non-identical BMT were thereafter made with the peculiar observation that none of the 12 patients thus treated rejected the partially-matched T-depleted marrow graft.[13,14] It was therefore proposed that lack of expression of LFA-1 by T and NK cells impaired the ability of host T and NK cells to reject donor marrow cells. Indeed in vitro allogeneic CTL as well as NK cell activities of LFA-1(-) lymphocytes were found to be strongly reduced.[12,15]

More recently, the C. Figdor's group has studied the ability of cattle with LAD to fully reject allogeneic skin grafts. They found in the 3 animals investigated a significant delay in graft-rejection, ranging from 12-14 days in controls to 28, 30 and 72 days respectively.[16] These data confirm and extend the concept that the LFA-1 molecule plays an important role in mediating interactions between rejection effector cells and target cells. Wilson et al have recently produced a CD18-mutant mouse with 2% on resting and 16% upon activation, normal CD18 surface expression by homologous recombination of the β2-CD18 encoding gene. H-2 incompatible heterotopic heart transplants were rejected after a significantly longer delay in these mice (16 days) as compared to control littermates (12 days).[17] Although the difference of magnitude is small, it again points to the role played by β2 integrins in graft rejection. Further experiments using a model of CD18 KO mice without β2 residual expression would be warranted to best define this role.

EXPERIMENTAL UTILIZATION OF ANTI-ADHESION ANTIBODIES IN ANIMAL MODELS

ANIMAL MODELS OF ANTI-ADHESION THERAPY

During the last 10 years, the efficacy of monoclonal antibodies specific for adhesion proteins, i.e. LFA-1, CD2, ICAM-1 and -3, LFA-3 to inhibit T and NK cell adhesion, activation and function has largely been demonstrated.[18-21] Additive effects of blocking both the LFA-1 and CD2 pathways have also been shown.[18,21] The concentration of antibodies required to observe a significant effect in vitro ranges to 10 µg/ml, a concentration that can easily be achieved in vivo. Blocking experiments were usually interpreted as inhibition of cell-to-cell interaction by steric hindrance of receptor/ligand binding. These many experiments taken together with the observations made with LFA-1(-) lymphocytes (see above) paved the way for the in vivo therapeutic use of monoclonal antibodies specific for adhesion molecules.

Heagy et al first injected anti-LFA-1 antibody to mice grafted with allogeneic tumors. They found that this antibody was a more potent inhibitor of tumor rejection than anti-CD8α or H-2 class I antibody or a mixture of all antibodies.[22]

From then onward, anti-LFA-1 antibody effects have been tested in several models of transplantation including marrow, heart, skin, pancreas islets and kidney (in monkeys) transplants. Antibodies specific for several other adhesion molecules (ICAM-1, CD2, VLA-4, VCAM-1) have also been investigated. The results of these transplants are summarized and discussed below.

MARROW

Van Dijken et al have shown that infusion of an anti-LFA-1 antibody (0.1 mg) for 5 days after injection of an H-2 incompatible T-depleted marrow preceded by an 11 Gray total body irradiation promotes marrow engraftment and leads to full immune reconstitution. This effect was marrow cell dose-dependent. If a

6×10^5 marrow cell dose was administered, survival rose from 5 to 20%, for a 2.5×10^6 marrow cell dose, survival rose from 40 to 85% and for 10×10^6 marrow cell dose, survival rose from 60 to 100%. 2.5×10^6 marrow cells/mouse correspond to $1.25/10^8$ cells/kg, a cell dose range commonly used in clinical BMT (see below).[23]

We found that in a haploidentical mouse combination, following a 9 Gray irradiation and injection of 2×10^6 T-depleted marrow cells, infusion of an anti-LFA-1 (CD11a) antibody at days - 1, 0, +1, +5, +7 and +9 (total dose 350 to 500 µg) improved the engraftment rate from 6 to 50% and survival of engrafted mice from 10 to 78%. Mice with mixed chimerism exhibited specific tolerance towards donor cells as neither alloreactive proliferation nor CTL activity could be generated in vitro against donor cells whereas reactivity to third party cells was preserved. In parallel, third party skin grafts where rejected while donor skin grafts were tolerated.[24]

Harning et al have explored the capacity of anti-LFA-1 antibody to treat acute GVHD in a P ' F1 transplant combination by infusing 10 mg/kg/day of the antibody for 10 days. They obtained a significant reduction in GVHD and prolongation of survival from 18 to 28 days. Similar use of an anti-ICAM-1 antibody had similar effects.[25]

HEART

Several groups have assessed the efficacy of anti-LFA-1 and/or anti-ICAM-1 antibodies to prevent rejection of allogeneic heterotopic heart transplants in mice.

The most impressive results were reported by Isobe et al who showed that an anti-LFA-1 Ab or an anti-ICAM-1 AB (alone) given each alone for 7 days (day 0 to +6, total dose of 300 µg) (or an anti-ICAM-1 Ab in the same way) had a mild effect in prolonging graft survival while 50 µg of both antibodies administered daily for six days promoted graft acceptance for more than 70 days, this in association with specific tolerance to donor alloantigens proven in vitro and in vivo.[26]

Other groups including ours did not obtain such striking results. However, here also significant effects brought by the use of any of those two Abs were reported.

We found that anti-LFA-1 antibody infusion (total dose 500 µg) from day -1 to +9 after an haploidentical vascularized heterotopic heart transplant, enhanced graft survival from 13 to 110 days.[24] In mice which did not reject heart transplants at day 70, host reactivity toward donor syngeneic cells could be shown in vitro (proliferation and CTL) as well as in vivo (skin graft).[24] It is noteworthy that the same regimen of anti-LFA-1 Ab administration did not delay rejection of haploidentical skin graft.

Nakakura et al showed that long term administration of an anti-LFA-1 Ab to recipients of allogeneic hearts (2 mg/kg/d for 20 days, then weekly up to day 96) led to a prolonged heart graft survival in 78% of the cases.[27]

In rats, Kameoka et al found a mild effect of anti-CD18 or ICAM-1 Ab administration on heterotopic heart graft survival, as survival was extended from 11 to 16 and 15 days respectively. Combined use of both Abs resulted in a 31-day mean survival[28] in one given combination of species whereas no effect was observed in another combination. In rat recipients of an allogeneic heterotopic heart graft, the injection of an anti-LFA-1 Ab for 13 days (total dose of 3,750 µg) extended heart survival from 7 to 24.5 days.[29] An anti-VLA-4 antibody also delayed heart rejection to 14.5 days. Combination of both antibodies did not improve the result obtained by anti-LFA-1 Ab alone.[29] Of note is the reduction by the use of those Abs of heart vasculitis 5 days post grafting.

Pelletier et al evaluated the efficacy of an anti-VCAM-1 antibody. They found an 80% rate of heart survival at day 21 versus 0% in a control group. Long term effects of the Ab were not reported.[30]

Interesting results were also obtained by studying the effects of anti-CD2 Ab injection over graft survival prolongation. However, it is more difficult to assess the in vivo effects of anti-CD2 antibody in mice as compared to humans since CD2 expression differs in both species, as well as in its overall function. Nevertheless, Qin et al showed that anti-CD2 administration after a heterotopic heart transplant at day 0 and +1 (200 µg total dose), prolonged survival from 13 to 24 days.[31] Injection in mice of an anti-CD48 antibody (CD48 is a CD2-ligand in mice but not in humans) prolonged survival to 20 days, while combination of both anti-CD48 and CD2 Abs promoted graft acceptance for at least 100 days, with conservation of CTL activity of host towards donor cells. It has been proposed that helper T-cell reactivity to donor was reduced. Of note is the observation of the profound modulation of CD2 expression[31] as also reported by Gückel et al.[32] Chavin et al also made similar observations concerning CD2.[33] They tested the possibility of synergism between the administration of a low dose of anti-CD2 antibody and immunosuppressive drugs. They obtained a synergistic effect by combining anti-CD2 antibody with a 60-day course of low dose of FK506, extending graft survival for over 165 days. Surprisingly, no similar effect was seen in either a combination with cyclosporine A or rapamycin.[33] Host anti-donor CTL reactivity was preserved and second donor syngeneic grafts were accepted.

Jendrisak et al tested the ability of a combination of anti-CD4, LFA-1 and ICAM-1 Abs to block rejection of allogeneic heterotopic heart transplants in mice. 15 µg of each antibody administered IP from day -3 to +10 prolonged graft survival from 15 to 59 days. This experimental protocol was based on previous in vitro data showing that this antibody combination could block mixed leukocyte reaction and induce anergy.[34]

PANCREAS ISLETS

Injection of anti-LFA-1 antibody showed a powerful immunosuppressive effect in allogeneic pancreas islet transplantation in mice. It resulted indeed in an indefinite survival of islets in 5/10 recipients with a mean survival time of 72 days versus 19 days in control mice. These results are impressive since antibody was injected at a dose of 100 µg at day 0 and +1 only. An anti-CD2 antibody had a more limited effect (mean survival 33 days) and a combination of anti-CD2 Ab with the anti-LFA-1 Ab did not improve survival as compared to the effect of the latter Ab alone.[35]

CORNEAL ALLOGRAFT

IP injection of anti-LFA-1 antibody (100 to 200 µg at days -2, -1, 0, +2, 4 and 7) reduced allogeneic corneal graft rejection from 90 to 47% of the mice grafted. Anti-ICAM-1 Ab did not produce a similar effect, even though (like the anti-LFA-1 Ab) it reduced CTL and delayed-type hypersensitivity (DTH) to donor antigens. Antibodies did not prevent rejection in preimmunized mice.[36]

Although it is difficult to draw firm conclusions from all of these experimental data mostly because of an heterogeneity either in the mice strains used for the production of the antibodies (epitope specificity and isotype), or in doses and frequency of administration, it is nevertheless clear that anti-adhesion molecules, especially those specific for LFA-1 and ICAM-1, can partially help prevent marrow and organ graft rejection. Synergistic effects between antibodies remain more difficult to assess at this time.

It is also obviously impossible to draw definitive conclusions regarding any possible clinical application since in many cases the doses of antibodies used largely exceed what can be therapeutically given to patients, and also knowing that molecule distribution and function can differ between mice and humans as demonstrated by CD2.

EXPERIMENTS IN MONKEYS

A single attempt at preventing kidney graft failure in sheep by infusion of an anti-LFA-1 antibody has been reported with an apparent ineffective result of the 0.125 mg/kg x 7 infusion administered.[37] In rhesus monkeys, interesting results have been provided regarding heart and kidney transplants. Cosimi et al found that injection of an anti-ICAM-1(R6-5-Bird) antibody at a dose of 1 or 2 mg/kg/day for 12 days was effective in preventing or treating graft rejection episodes. Although the effect was not long-lasting, the authors concluded that anti-ICAM-1 Ab alone had a very efficient immunosuppressive effect in this setting. Interestingly enough, antibody infusion did not prevent infiltration of donor kidney by leukocytes although they appeared not harmful.[38] Similarly, Flavin et al using the same MoAb extended heart allograft survival in cynomologous monkeys from 8 to 23 or 26 days by injecting 1 to 2 mg/kg/day from day -2 to +10 (in cynomologous monkeys).[39]

In the same species, Berlin et al assessed the consequences of anti-LFA-1 or -CD2 specific monoclonal Ab section. A 10-day course of 0.5 to 1 mg/kg/day of either antibody led to:

1. generation of anti-mouse Ig antibodies with both idiotypic and non idiotypic specificities;
2. lack of T-cell depletion;
3. modulation of LFA-1 but not of CD2 molecule expression (in contrast to data in mice); and
4. mild prolongation in skin allografts by anti-LFA-1 Ab but not by the anti-CD2 Ab.[40]

These pre-clinical results provide important information on the efficacy and the limit of use of these antibodies.

CLINICAL USE OF ANTI-ADHESION ANTIBODIES

MARROW

We initiated the administration of anti-LFA-1 (CD11a) antibody in children recipients of T-depleted HLA partially incompatible marrow transplants for inherited diseases. The rationale was based on clinical observations in patients with LAD (see above) as well as the known in vitro immunosuppressive effects of anti-LFA-1 Ab.[1,2] A first open multicenter trial showed that infusion of 0.1 mg/kg of 25/3 anti-LFA-1 MoAb (IgG1) at days -3 to +5 (every other day), though partially clinically efficient in preventing graft-rejection and non-toxic, led to low to undetectable trough serum levels of the Ab.[41,42] It was therefore decided to infuse anti-LFA-1 Ab daily from day -3 to +6 at a dose of 0.2 mg/kg, a therapeutic scheme that gave very promising clinical results. Whereas, in a control historical group of children with inherited disorders including primary immunodeficiencies excluding SCID and osteopetrosis patients, engraftment rate was 25% with a long term survival of 8% (n = 24) in the group of patients receiving the Ab, the engraftment rate was 72% and long term survival 45%[43] (n = 42). This shows significant, even if partial, effect of anti-LFA-1 antibody infusion in recipients of haploidentical T-cell depleted marrows. Apart from anti-LFA-1 Ab infusion, control and study groups had similar characteristics. Also, no side effects due to AB administration were recorded and patients did not develop anti-mouse Ig antibodies (HAMA).

Pharmacokinetic studies showed a gradual accumulation of antibody in the serum with trough) serum levels ≥ 1 μg/ml from day 0.[42] In vitro, the same concentration of antibody had significant inhibitory activity (in vitro) on T-cell proliferation and cytotoxicity.

In order to try to improve engraftment rate in this clinical setting by further blocking lymphocyte adhesion, a second open multicenter trial was designed in which patients received administration of the anti-LFA-1 Ab from day -3 to +10 in combination with a monoclonal murine IgG2b specific for CD2 (B-E2). In this study, it appeared that results differed according to the method of T-cell depletion used. In recipients of E-rosette depleted marrow engraftment rate was 81% and survival 58.3% versus 68.8% and 43.8% respectively in the historical control group treated by anti-

LFA-1 Ab only.[44] Possibly, a trend towards improvement of engraftment has thus been obtained but this needs to be confirmed by further controlled evaluation. However, in recipients of a Campath-1M T-depleted marrow, results were less satisfactory with a 20% engraftment rate, this likely because of a more reduced number of T-cells infused with the marrow cells, and possible depletion of other cell-types required for engraftment.

Anti-LFA-1 + anti-CD2 Ab have also been administered in children with high-risk acute lymphoblastic leukemia who lacked an HLA genetically identical donor. Patients above age 2 were fractioned TBI (12 Gray), Aracytine (12 g/m²) and Melphalan (140 mg/m²). Marrow was T-cell-depleted using anti-CD2 and anti-CD7 Abs. The Engraftment rate was 80% among the 24 children thus treated, confirming the efficacy of these antibodies in promoting engraftment. After 2 years, disease-free survival is 40% (after 2 years) while event-free survival is 29%. The residual but serious problem of haplo-identical BMT in these settings consists in the long lasting T-cell immunodeficiency likely caused by marrow T-cell depletion (not by LFA-1- and CD2-specific antibody that are not depleting) which results in a high mortality rate through severe infections and leukemia relapse.[45]

A therapeutic trial using anti-LFA-1 Ab was also tested (anti-CD18) in adults receiving a T-depleted haplo-identical BMT. It had no detectable effect in preventing graft rejection.[46] Discrepancy could be accounted for either by use of a distinct Ab or more likely by insufficient cell inoculum. As shown by Van Dijken et al[23] (see above), the protective effect in mice of anti-LFA-1 antibody is dependent on the marrow cell dose.

Anti-LFA-1 antibody has also been used with some success to treat steroid-resistant GVHD,[47,48] although it appeared that any beneficial effect obtained could only be transient.

KIDNEY TRANSPLANTATION

The same 25/3 antibody has first been used to try to treat rejection episodes of kidney grafts in seven patients. Antibody administration failed to reverse rejection. It was noticed that immunization to 25/3 was infrequent and weak.[49]

With the aim of preventing rather than treating kidney graft rejection, a pilot study using the 25/3 Ab in 15 patients was undertaken.[50] Decreasing doses of 20, 15 and 10 mg/patient/day were given for 2 weeks in conjunction with cyclosporine A (from day 9), steroids and azathioprine. Trough serum levels above 10 μg/ml were achieved with saturation of targets and modulation of expression. Delayed graft function lasted 8 ± 6 days. Frequency of rejection episodes was 6 in 14 evaluable patients in the first 3 months and they were reversible under treatment. Thus the antibody appeared promising for preventing early rejection and was not associated with severe side effects. Immunization occurred in half of the patients.

These results were judged promising enough to warrant a controlled randomized trial (presently ongoing), comparing anti-LFA-1 Ab to ATG in the prevention of kidney graft rejection.

In this regard, Cosimi's group designed a pilot study evaluating the possible efficacy of an anti-ICAM-1 antibody in preventing kidney graft rejection following the positive results obtained in monkeys (see above). Eighteen patients with a high risk of acute graft rejection (because of prolonged preservation time or highly sensitized patient) were included. Increasing doses of anti-ICAM-1 Ab were given beginning with a 20 mg initial dose followed by 10 mg for 14 days, up to 160 mg initial dose followed by 80 mg/5 days, this in order to adjust serum level above 10 mg/ml.[51] Patients with serum concentration ≥ 10 μg/ml had less rejection episodes. Taken together, 78% of grafts were functional 16 to 30 months post transplantation versus 56% of contralateral kidneys transplanted in a non controlled group which received conventional immunosuppression.[51]

Here again, the results were promising enough to launch a controlled randomized phase III trial (presently ongoing). It is thought that anti-ICAM-1 antibody acts through an inhibition of leukocyte/endothelial cell interaction. Of note is the lack of any side effects of antibody infusion despite HAMA occurrence in 16/18 patients.

At this writing, we are not aware of any other reports of a clinical study using anti-adhesion molecules antibodies in the transplantation setting; it is likely, however, that several others involving liver, heart and possibly gut transplantation are scheduled.

MECHANISM OF ACTION

We have reviewed a large set of experimental and clinical data which indicate that anti-adhesion molecule antibodies can exert effective immunosuppression with limited toxicity.

Several possible mechanisms can account for these effects. Cell depletion can be excluded for several reasons: None of the antibodies used bind complement and they do not appear to induce neither antibody mediated cytotoxicity nor phagocytosis. Many (but not all) of these antibodies have a murine IgG1 isotype associated with poor binding to human Fc γ receptors. More importantly, it was observed in many studies including clinical studies with LFA-1- and ICAM-1-specific antibodies that none of them induced blood leukocyte depletion.[42,49-51]

Since antibodies were not depleted, inhibition of function was postulated. Modulation of expression, shown for CD2 in mice and LFA-1 in humans,[31,42,50] can partially account for lack of adhesion receptor function. In any case, modulation is partial (by a factor of 2 or 3) and thus is not sufficient by itself to account for immunosuppression.

Therefore, steric hindrance of receptor/ligand interaction is the most likely explanation. That in some instance, simultaneous blockade of receptor and ligand (LFA-1/ICAM-1, CD2/CD48 in mice) reinforced immunosuppression, (is in) favor (of) this hypothesis (provided that each antibody was not saturating). Steric hindrance may explain suppression of NK and T-cell responses and blockade of leukocyte migration by inhibition of leukocyte/endothelial cell interaction.

The most fascinating question deals with persistence of specific immunosuppression observed in many models following administration of anti-adhesion antibodies. This effect was partially observed in allogeneic heart transplants and islet transplants in mice as well as in marrow transplantation in mice and humans. It appears mainly associated with the use of anti-LFA-1 antibody.[24,26,28,35,43,44]

How could a short-term infusion of antibody prevent rejection for many weeks in these settings? There is no clear mechanism to account for these observations. Induction of tolerance, possibly by anergy, is an attractive hypothesis. Benjamin et al have shown that immunization of mice with human IgG did not lead to antibody production in mice receiving simultaneous infusion of an anti-LFA-1 antibody (or anti-CD4).[52] That immunization in humans against murine anti-LFA-1 Ab, although present, appears slightly less frequent and intense as compared with anti-CD3 and/or anti-IL2R antibody administration, might therefore also point to a similar phenomenon.

There are controversial data concerning defective in vitro as well as in vivo helper and CTL activity of host T-cells towards donor cells in mice transplanted under the "umbrella" of anti-LFA-1 Ab.[24,26-29] In some reports CTL are abolished or reduced, while in others they are not. More careful work will obviously be needed to sort out this question. One may however speculate that antigen (alloantigen) administration in the presence of anti T-cell adhesion molecules may prevent full activation, i.e., signals "1" and "2" respectively given by the T-cell receptor and CD28.[53] One may propose that adhesion molecules (LFA-1, CD2, ICAM-3) can either directly or indirectly participate in signal 2 reception and transmission. If this hypothesis is correct, anti-adhesion molecule antibodies could somehow act as blocking agents of the CD28/CD80 pathway as CTLA-4 Ig does.[54] It would be of great interest to combine in vivo these two approaches in order to have additive and possibly synergistic effects.

It is also possible that binding of anti-adhesion molecules to their targets induces signaling repressing cell activation as postulated in models of in vitro inhibitory effects of anti-CD4 Ab.[55] Chavin et al have shown that in vivo immunosuppressive effects mediated by anti-CD2 Ab in mice can be transferred by T-cells since CD4 T-cells were able to suppress CTL reactivity. These CD4 cells exhibit a "TH2" phenotype with production of IL-4 and TGF β.[56,57] This effect is in part reminiscent of infectious tolerance achieved by an in vivo infusion of anti-CD4 antibody in mice.[58]

Although the long-lasting immunosuppressive effect of anti-adhesion molecules is somewhat limited, there is considerable interest in their potential application. It will be necessary to develop models to study the molecular mechanism of action to promote the design of further immunosuppressive strategies.

ACKNOWLEDGMENTS
This work was supported by grants from INSERM and ARC.

REFERENCES
1. Springer TA. Adhesion receptors of the immune system. Nature 1990; 346:425-434.
2. Hyners RO. Integrins: versatility, modulation and signaling in cell adhesion. Cell 1992; 69:11-25.
3. Diamond MS, Springer TA. The dynamic regulation of integrin

adhesiveness. Current Biol 1994; 4:506-517.

4. Amblard F, Auffray C, Sekaly R et al. Molecular analysis of anti-gen-independent adhesion forces between T and B lymphocytes. PNAS 1994; 91:3628-3632.

5. Fischer A. Anti-LFA-1 antibody as immunosuppressive reagent in transplantation. Chem Immunol 1991; 50:89-97.

6a. Landis RC, McDowall A, Holness CLL et al. Involvement of the "I" domain of LFA-1 in selective binding to ligands ICAM-1 to ligands ICAM-1 and ICAM-3. J Cell Biol 1994; 126:529-537.

6b. Stanley P, Bastes PA, Harvey JA et al. Integrin LFA-1 a subunit contains an ICAM-1 binding site in domains V and VI. Embo J 1994; 13:1790-1798.

7. Dustin Ml, Springer TA. T-cell receptor cross-linking transiently stimulates adhesiveness through LFA-1. Nature 1989; 341:619-621.

8. Van Kooyk Y, Van De Wiel-Van Kemenade E, Weder P et al. Enhancement of LFA-1-mediated cell adhesion by triggering through CD2 or CD3 on T-lymphocytes. Nature 1989; 342:811-13.

9. Arroyo AG, Campanero MR, Sanchez-Mateos P et al. Induction of tyrosine phosphorylation during ICAM-3 and LFA-1 mediated intercellular adhesion and its regulation by the CD45 tyrosine phosphatase. J Cell Biol 1994; 126:1277-1286.

10. Van Seventer GA, Shimizu Y, Horgan KJ et al. The LFA-1 ligand ICAM-1 provides an important costimulary signal for T-cell receptor-mediated activation of resting T-cells. J Immunol 1990; 144:4579-4583.

11. Figdor CG, Van Kooyk Y, Keizer GD. On the mode of action of LFA-1. Immunol Today 1950; 11:277-279.

12. Fischer A, Lisowska-Grospierre B, Anderson DC et al. The leukocyte adhesion deficiency. Immunodef Rev 1988; 2:39-54.

13. Le Deist F, Blanche S, Keable H et al. Successful HLA-non identical bone marrow transplantation in three patients with leukocyte adhesion deficiency. Blood 1989; 74:512-517.

14. Thomas C, Le Deist F, Friedrich W et al. Bone marrow transplantation for the treatment of children with leukocyte adhesion deficiency. A revue of 14 cases. Submitted.

15. Kohl S, Loo Ls, Schmalstieg FS et al. The genetic deficiency of leukocyte surface glycoproteins Mac-1, LFA-1, p150,95 in humans is associated with defective antibody-dependent cellular cytotoxicity and defective protection against herpes simplex virus infection in vivo. J Immunol 1986; 177:1688-1693.

16. Muller KE, Rutten UPMG, Becker CK et al. Skin transplantations in β2-integrin deficient cattle.

17. Wilson RW, Ballatyne CM, Smith CW et al. Gene targeting yields a CD18-mutant mouse for study of inflammation. J Immunol 1993; 151:1571-1578.

18. Makgoba MW, Sangers ME, Shaw S. The CD2/LFA-3 and LFA-

1/ICAM pathways: relevance to T-cell recognition. Immunol Today 1989; 10:417-420.

19. Krensky AM, Sanchez-Madrid F, Robbins E et al. The functional significance, distribution and structure of LFA-1, LFA-2 and LFA-3: cell surface antigens associated with CTL-target interactions. J Immunol 1983; 131:611-617.

20. Mentzer SJ, Krensky AM, Burakoff SJ. Mapping functional epitopes of the human LFA-1 glycoprotein: monoclonal antibody inhibition of NK and CTL effectors. Hum Immunol 1986; 17:288-295.

21. Mazerolles F, Lumbroso C, Lecomte O et al. The role of LFA-1 in the adherence of T-lymphocytes to B-lymphocytes. Eur J Immunol 1988; 18:1229-1234.

22. Heagy W, Waltenbaugh C. Potent ability of anti-LFA-1 monoclonal antibody to prolong allograft survival. Transplantation 1984; 37:520-523.

23. Van Dijken PJ, Ghayur T, Mauch P et al. Evidence that anti-LFA-1 in vivo improves engraftment and survival after allogeneic bone marrow transplantation. Transplantation 1990; 49:882-886.

24. Cavazzaana-Calvo M, Sarnacki S, Haddad E et al. Prevention of bone marrow and cardiac graft rejection in an H-2 haplotype disparate mouse combination by an anti-LFA-1 antibody. Submitted.

25. Harning R, Pelletier J, Lubbe K et al. Reduction in the severity of graft-versus host disease and increased survival in allogeneic mice by treatment with monoclonal antibodies to cell adhesion antigens LFA-1a and MALA-2. Transplantation 1991; 52:842-845.

26. Isobe M, Yagita H, Okumura K et al. Specific acceptance of cardiac allograft after treatment with antibodies to ICAM-1 and LFA-1. Science 1992; 255:1125-1127.

27. Nakakura EK, McCabe SM, Zheng B et al. Potent and effective prolongation by anti-LFA-1 monoclonal antibody monotherapy of non-primarily vascularized heart allograft survival in mice without T-cell depletion. Transplantation 1993; 55:412-417.

28. Kameoka H, Ishibashi M, Tamantani T et al. The immunosuppressive action of anti-CD18 monoclonal antibody in rat heterotopic heart allotransplantation. Transplantation 1993; 55:665-667.

29. Paul LC, Davidoff A, Benediktsson M et al. The efficacy of LFA-1 and VLA-4 antibody treatment in rat vascularized cardiac allograft rejection. Transplantation 1993; 55:1196-1199.

30. Pelletier R, Ohye R, Kincade P et al. Monoclonal antibody to anti-VCAM-1 interferes with murine cardiac allograft rejection. Transplant Proc 1993; 25:839-841.

31. Qin L, Chavin KD, Lin J et al. Anti-CD2 receptor and anti-CD2 ligand (CD48) antibodies synergize to prolong allograft survival. J Exp Med 1994; 179:341-346.

32. Gückel B, Berek C, Lutz M, Altevogt P et al. Anti-CD2 antibodies induce T-cell unresponsiveness in vivo. J Exp Med 1991;

174:957-967.

33. Chavin K, Qin L, Woodward JE et al. Anti-CD2 monoclonal antibodies synergize with FK506 but not with cyclosporine or rapamycin to induce tolerance. Transplantation 1994; 57:736-740.

34. Jendrisak M, Jendrisak G, Gamero J et al. Prolongation in murine cardiac survival with monoclonal antibodies to LFA-1, ICAM-1 and CD4. Transplant Proc 1993; 25:825-827.

35. Gotoh M, Fukuzaki T, Mondren M et al. A potential immunosuppressive effect of anti-lymphocyte function-associated antigen-1 monoclonal antibody on islet transplantation. Transplantation 1994; 57:123-126.

36. He YG, Mellon J, Apte R et al. Effect of LFA-1 and ICAM-1 antibody treatment on murine corneal allograft survival. Invest Ophtalmol Vis Sci 1994; 35:3218-3225;

37. Grooby WL, Carter JK, Rao MM et al. Use of an anti-LFA-1 antibody in renal allograft rejection in sheep. Transplant Proc 1992; 24:2304.

38. Cosimi AB, Conti D, Delmonico FL et al. In vivo effects of monoclonal antibody to ICAM-1 (CD54) in non human primates with renal allografts. J Immunol 1990; 144:4604-4612.

39. Flavin T, Ivens K, Faanes R et al. Monoclonal antibodies against IC AM-1 prolony cardic allograft survival in cynomolgus monkeys. Transplant Proc 1991; 23:533-534.

40. Berlin PJ, Bacher JD, Sharrow SO et al. Monoclonal antibodies against human T-cell adhesion molecules—modulation of immune function in non human primates. Transplantation 1992; 53:840-849.

41. Fischer A, Blanche S, Veber F et al. Prevention of graft failure by an anti-LFA-1 monoclonal antibody in HLA mismatched bone marrow transplantation. Lancet 1986; 2:1068-1071.

42. Perez N, Le Deist F, Chatenoud L et al. In vivo infusions of anti-LFA-1 antibody in HLA non identical and biological effects. Bone Marrow Transplant 1989; 4:379-385.

43. Fischer A, Friedrich W, Fasth A et al. Reduction of graft failure by a monoclonal antibody (anti-LFA-1, CD11a) after HLA-non identical bone marrow transplantation in children with immunodeficiencies, osteopetrosis and Fanconi's anemia. Blood 1991; 2:249-256.

44. Jabado N, Le Deist F, De Graaf Meiders B et al. Combined use of two monoclonal antibodies (anti-LFA-1 and anti-CD2) to prevent graft rejection in recipients of T-depleted marrow from genetically HLA-non identical donors in children with inherited disorders. Submitted.

45. Cavazzana-Calvo M, Bordigoni P, Michel G, Baruchel A et al. Partially incompatible marrow transplantation therapy for high risk acute lymphoblastic leukemia in children: Analysis of prevention of graft rejection by anti-LFA-1 and anti-CD2 antibodies. A SFGM

study. Submitted.

46. Baume D, Kuentz M, Pico JL et al. Failure of a CD18/anti-LFA-1 monoclonal antibody infusion to prevent graft rejection in leukemic patients receiving T-depleted allogeneic bone marrow transplantation. Transplantation 1989; 47:472-474.

47. Marawinchi D, Mawas C, Stoppa AM et al. Anti-LFA-1 monoclonal antibody for the prevention of graft rejection after T-cell depleted HLA-matched bone marrow transplantation for leukemia in adults. Bone Marrow Transplant 1989; 4:147.

48. Ohashi Y, Tsuchiya S, Fujie H et al. Anti-LFA-1 antibody treatment of a patient with steroid-resistant severe graft-versus-host disease. Tohoku J Exp Med 1992; 167:297-299.

49. Le Mauff B, Hourmant M, Rougier JP et al. Effect of anti-LFA-1 (CD11a) monoclonal antibodies in acute rejection in human kidney transplantation. Transplantation 1991; 52:291-296.

50. Hourmant M. Le Mauff B, Le Meur Y et al. Administration of an anti-CD11a monoclonal antibody in recipients of kidney transplantation. A pilot study. Transplantation 1994; 58:377-380.

51. Haugg CE, Colvin RB, Delmonico FL et al. A phase I trial of immunosuppression with ICAM-1 (CD54) MoAb in renal allograft recipients. Transplantation 1993; 55:766-773.

52. Benjamin RJ, Qui S, Wise MP et al. Mechanisms of monoclonal antibody-facilitated tolerance induction: a possible role for the CD4 (L3T4) and CD11a (LFA-1) molecules in self-non-self discrimination. Eur J Immunol 1988; 18:1079-84.

53. Schwartz RH. A cell culture model for T lymphocyte clonal anergy. Science 1990; 248:1349-1356.

54. Wallace PM, Johnson JS, MacMaster JF et al. CTLA4 Ig treatment ameliorates the lethality of murine graft-versus-host disease across major histocompatibility complex barriers. Transplantation 1994; 58:602-610.

55. Janeway CA, Carding S, Jones B et al. CD4[+] T-cells: specificity and function. Immunol Rev 1988; 101:39-80.

56. Chavin KD, Qin L, Yon R et al. Anti-CD2 MoAbs suppress cytotoxic lymphocytic activity by the generation of Th2 suppressor cells and receptor blockade. J Immunol 1994; 152:3729-3739.

57. Ohno H, Nakamura T, Yagita H et al. Induction of negative signal through CD2 during antigen-specific T-cell activation. J Immunol 1991; 147:2100-2106.

58. Qin S, Cobbold SP, Pope H et al. "Infectious tolerance" transplantation tolerance. Science 1993; 259:974-977.

CHAPTER 6

FUTURE GOALS FOR THERAPEUTIC MONOCLONAL ANTIBODIES

Lucienne Chatenoud, Michelle Webb and Jean-François Bach

INTRODUCTION

Fifteen years of experience in using immunosuppressive mono-clonal antibodies for studies predominantly in experimental and clinical transplantation, but also in autoimmunity, has clearly demonstrated the existence of therapeutic activities not shared by conventional chemical immunosuppressants (i.e. corticosteroids, azathioprine, cyclosporine, FK506). Antibodies to CD3 (OKT3) have been remarkably efficacious in reversing severe acute allograft rejection, a clinical situation in which only high-dose steroids and polyclonal antilymphocyte antibodies have similar efficacy.[1-3] More importantly, antibodies or genetically engineered molecules to distinct T-cell receptors (CD4, CD4+CD8, CD28/CTLA4Ig, adhesion receptors or adhesins) can promote tolerance, namely, a stable and antigen-specific state of immunological unresponsiveness.[4] As a result, a wide variety of experimental situations have been described where T cell-directed monoclonal antibodies have afforded tolerance not only to foreign soluble antigens but also to tissue alloantigens and autoantigens.[5-16] Thus, despite the different problems surrounding their production and clinical development, i.e.

Monoclonal Antibodies in Transplantation, edited by Lucienne Chatenoud. © 1995 R.G. Landes Company.

high cost and side effects (namely, acute cytokine-related syndrome, xenosensitization), continued effort in pursuing the study of therapeutic monoclonals appears worthwhile.

Imagine if one could achieve specific tolerance in clinical organ transplantation? At one fell swoop one would avoid the two major hazards of chronic immunosuppressive therapy, namely, its relative long term ineffectiveness with consequent recurrence of the destructive immunopathologic processes, and the well documented infectious and tumorigenic risks. Obviating the need for chronic immunosuppression would allow the extension of monoclonal antibody use to immune-mediated clinical disorders other than allograft rejection, in particular, to autoimmune diseases. Moreover, from a more fundamental point of view, an understanding of the molecular basis of the tolerogenic properties of monoclonal antibodies would clear the way for development of more easily accessible therapeutic strategies i.e., simple chemicals or recombinant receptor agonist and/or antagonist ligands that would mimic the desired therapeutic effect. This need is further supported by the wealth of data showing that antibodies express unique pharmacological activities. For instance, naturally occurring (i.e. spontaneous autoimmunity) anti-receptor antibodies may either block receptor function (anti-acetylcholine receptor antibodies or anti-insulin receptor antibodies)[17] or express clear-cut agonistic properties (anti-thyroid stimulating hormone receptor antibodies).[17] The real challenge for the future for both immunologists and pharmacologists, will be to dissect the molecular and cellular mechanisms through which antibodies express these subtle modulatory effects.

ANTIBODIES TO T-CELL RECEPTORS AS UNIQUE TOLERANCE-PROMOTING TOOLS

Achieving donor-specific tolerance while preserving normal immune responsiveness to other foreign antigens is a major goal in clinical transplantation. The first observations of a state of immune tolerance to allogeneic cells was made by R. Owen. He reported that cattle dizygotic twins born from a common placenta maintained, throughout life, allogeneic circulating cells from each other.[18] Skin grafts performed between such twins, whom were lymphohemopoietic chimeras, were retained indefinitely. Some years later in 1953, the experiments of R. Billingham, L. Brent and P. Medawar proved for the first time that immunological tolerance to alloantigens could be acquired.[19] In their original experiments these authors showed that neonatal mice injected within 24 h from delivery with allogeneic cells, as adults, indefinitely accepted skin grafts sharing the same haplotype as the cells injected at birth. This tolerant state was specific since the animals could reject third party allogeneic skin. When bone marrow was used as a source of tolerogen, a low proportion of donor cells, i.e. microchimerism, persisted throughout life in tolerant recipients.

Although, for obvious reasons, these models did not have direct clinical application, they have been an extremely rich source of fundamental information needed to undertake the first tentative experiments aim at tolerance induction in adult animals. These initial studies also demonstrated that successful induction of stable lymphohemopoietic mixed chimerism is a potent means of inducing robust specific transplantation tolerance to solid organs across major histocompatibility barriers thus implying that bone marrow is a privileged source of tolerogenic alloantigens.[20]

For many years the question central to the debate has been whether antigen-specific unresponsiveness is due to selective deletion of T cells specific for the inoculated alloantigens from the recipients' T cell repertoire or to a functional inhibition of such alloreactive cells. The experimental evidence suggests that both mechanisms could coexist to varying degrees depending on the inherent parameters of the experimental system. This includes the intrinsic characteristics of the alloantigen used as a tolerogen.[21-27]

Thus, animals tolerized at birth show a significantly decreased frequency of alloreactive T-cell precursors, however, they are not completely eliminated. This clonal deletion can be demonstrated at the structural level using Vβ-specific monoclonal antibodies.[27] Alternatively, supporting the thesis of cell-mediated immunoregulatory mechanisms sustaining unresponsiveness is data showing that the tolerant state cannot be reversed by the infusion of nontolerant host-type lymphocytes and that lymphoid cells from neonatally-treated animals can transfer tolerance to adult syngeneic recipients.[21] Studies performed in a rat model suggest that a host-type cell subset staining CD4+CD45+ and showing anti-idiotypic specificity (i.e. the suppressor cells specifically recognize determinants of the TCR of donor-reactive T cells) is responsible for the transfer capacity and the "resistance" to breaking of tolerance.[21] In this model, lymphohemopoietic chimerism was found to be essential for the maintenance of tolerance; persistent donor-type cells were required for the adoptive transfer of tolerance although they were not the effectors of suppression. One possibility is that donor antigen acts as a permanent stimulus for the generation of idiotypic and hence of anti-idiotypic cells. Alternatively, hemopoietic cells may provide a unique and persistent source of deleting antigen.

Over the last 20 years major efforts have been devoted to recreating in the adult host the same "permissive" environment for transplantation as that present in the immunologically immature neonate.

Most strategies have involved immunosuppression delivered in association with alloantigen exposure, but have differed in the source of alloantigen (bone marrow, whole blood or the allograft itself), the nature of the immunosuppressive treatment and the kinetics within a given protocol.

Promoting stable lymphohemopoietic mixed chimerism following allogeneic bone marrow transplantation currently necessitates the use of myeloablative protocols.[20,28,29] Substantial bone marrow engraftment requires "conditioning" of the recipient to both create hematopoietic "space" and reduce "alloresistance." This elusive and poorly understood concept of "space" is of major practical concern in that optimal engraftment, not only of allogeneic but also of syngeneic bone marrow, can only be achieved by deleting part of the recipients' lymphohemopoietic system.[30,31] It is important to stress that creating space does not necessarily imply the use of an immunosuppressive treatment[30,31] although most conditioning regimens (i.e. irradiation) are effective in doing both.

In contrast, "alloresistance" is of concern only in cases of allogeneic bone marrow transplantation. It involves in the main T-cell-mediated mechanisms and dictates the need for strong immunosuppresive treatment as part of host conditioning. Such myeloablative methods used to create mixed allogeneic chimeras in mice require the use of fairly toxic treatments (e.g. lethal whole body irradiation) which could never be justifiable for the purpose of organ transplantation.[28,32] These types of protocols are used exclusively for bone marrow transplantation in the context of treating hematological malignancies, a situation in which whole body irradiation is given in combination with chemotherapy. The degree of immunocompetence induced in the recipient by this type of strategy negates its use in clinical organ transplantation.

The approach holding perhaps the greatest promise for the foreseeable future involves the use of non-myeloablative conditioning regimens. In particular those involving exclusive administration of either polyclonal or monoclonal antibodies to eliminate host elements resisting marrow engraftment, and using as a source of alloantigen, bone marrow or blood transfusion in conjunction with the organ allograft.

The early pioneers in transplantation, in the absence of the development of monoclonal antibodies against specific components of the immune system, attempted to attain tolerance using rather aggressive broad spectrum immunosuppressive protocols. Monaco and Wood's ground-breaking experiments in the 1960s[33,34] used a combination of anti-lymphocyte serum (ALS) treatment and post-transplantation donor bone marrow infusion to induce specific unresponsiveness to C3H/He skin allografts in (C57BL6 x A/J)F1 (B6AF1) mice.[33,34] Although in this model skin graft survival was significantly prolonged, indefinite engraftment was seldom attained. Thymectomising adult mice prior to ALS treatment, and post-transplant donor bone marrow infusion, significantly prolonged skin graft survival (90% of the grafts surviving over 100 days and 40% permanently). The effect was specific since third party grafts were rapidly rejected and lymphohemopoietic microchimerism was observed in tolerant animals. Suppressor T cells have been implicated in the specific unresponsiveness observed in these animals.[35]

Interestingly, recent data suggest that rapamycin, used at doses that are ineffective on their own in promoting skin graft survival, can successfully replace adult thymectomy.[36]

It has been reported that rapamycin, in addition to preventing the maturation and proliferation of IL-2 receptor expressing committed cells, causes significant depletion of both the thymic cortex and medulla. This depletion is primarily one of double positive $CD4^+CD8^+$ cells, and continues long beyond the end of treatment.

Monaco's results were important since they demonstrated for the first time that it was possible to manipulate the allogeneic response of an adult host and prolong organ allograft survival. In addition, the results indicated that the degree of difficulty in achieving tolerance was directly correlated to H-2 disparity between the donor and the recipient, thus needing careful adaptation of the induction protocol; in particular the lag time between ALS administration and bone marrow. This needed to be sufficiently short to maintain immunosuppression at the time of bone marrow delivery, but sufficiently long to avoid destruction of bone marrow cells by free circulating ALS.[33,34]

This approach, with modifications, has been successfully used to transplant mismatched renal allograft in non-human primates. Prolonged survival of histoincompatible kidney transplants has been achieved in rhesus monkeys with a combination of rabbit anti-thymocyte globulin (ATG) and a post-transplantation donor bone marrow infusion.[37-40] However, the best results have been obtained with combined ATG and total lymphoid irradiation (TLI) induction therapy followed by a post-transplant infusion of bone marrow depleted of bright CD3+/DR+ cells.[39-40] Studies aimed at characterizing the cells promoting long term engraftment in these experiments have identified a small fraction of the bone marrow population which stain CD2+ CD8+ CD16+ DR- CD3- CD38- and whose in vitro behavior corresponds with the classical definition of veto cells i.e. an aberrant antigen-presenting cell that inactivates CTL precursor clones by providing a negative, possibly deleting, signal.[41] The unresponsiveness generated was specific for the donor alloantigens. Microchimerism was demonstrated by the polymerase chain reaction (PCR), in both non-rejecting and rejecting recipients. The infusion of allogeneic bone marrow was perfectly well tolerated and elicited neither sensitization nor graft versus host disease.[37-40]

Following the development of anti-T-cell monoclonal antibodies, it has become apparent that some have unique tolerogenic capacities, in particular, antibodies to CD4. The first important finding was that rat anti-CD4 injected into mice did not trigger antiglobulin response as was the case with other rodent monoclonal antibodies against different T-cell antigens.[5,6]

The effect was dose-dependent, low doses, as opposed to high doses, being immunogenic. High-dose anti-CD4-treated mice remained unresponsive upon rechallenge with the same monoclonal antibody while reacting fully towards third party antigens, indicating the induction of a specific tolerance state.[5,6] It has been subsequently shown that delivering soluble antigens under the cover of anti-CD4 monoclonal antibodies induced specific tolerance to the foreign soluble proteins, i.e. human γ globulins. Neither the antigen nor the monoclonal antibody alone were sufficient to elicit this tolerance and both had to be delivered within a limited period of time.[5,6,42-46] Depletion of CD4⁺ cells was irrelevant in achieving this effect. Tolerance could also be induced with F(ab')2 fragments or non-depleting monoclonal antibody isotypes (for instance rat IgG2a in mice).[47,48] Importantly, all that was needed to maintain tolerance in normal euthymic animals was the antigen alone, delivered at regular time intervals, in the absence of any further monoclonal antibody treatment. If mice tolerant to human γ globulins were left without further antigen challenge for over four months they recovered their ability to respond.[5,6] The same strategy, i.e., delivering a single high dose anti-CD4 injection in association with ordinarily immunogenic therapeutic molecules, has been successfully used in rodents to prevent deleterious sensitization against various xenogeneic monoclonal antibodies including anti-CD3.[44,49]

H. Waldmann's group was the first to demonstrate that some monoclonal antibodies, in particular combinations of antibodies to CD4 and CD8, could induce classical transplantation tolerance. Specific tolerance to skin grafts was achieved in mice across a multiple minor or a class I and multiple minor histocompatibility barrier by using combined antibodies to CD4 and CD8 together with bone marrow engraftment (microchimerism: 1-5% donor blood cells).[50] In this model T-cell-depleted bone marrow was used to avoid the potential risk of graft versus host disease. Skin allografts from the bone marrow donor strain could be implanted any time from the day of bone marrow infusion to more than 300 days later and still result in permanent engraftment, whereas third-party skin allografts were rapidly rejected.[50] No evidence for clonal deletion of specific alloreactive T cells was found in these models, but in some cases anergy was demonstrated i.e. in vitro unresponsiveness to the donor alloantigen while the sensitivity to anti-TCR driven stimulation is kept.[50]

The next step forward was the demonstration that tolerance to skin grafts could be induced, without the need for marrow infusions. Adult thymectomized CBA/Ca mice were transplanted with skin from B10.BR (minor-histocompatibility mismatch) under the cover of combined non-depleting (IgG2a) antibodies to CD4 and CD8 (0.5mg each applied at days 0, 2 and 4 after skin grafting).[7,48,51,52] Injection of fresh naive CBA/Ca, together with fresh B10.BR grafts, could not break the tolerance, a phenomenon termed "resistance." Second skin grafts from the original donor were accepted indefinitely. Moreover, CD4⁺ cells from tolerant animals could mediate suppression of naive lymphocytes upon conventional adoptive transfer.[51] Importantly, by injecting the naïve T cells into tolerant recipients transgenic for human CD2 it was possible to show that an in vivo coexistence of about two weeks was necessary to render them tolerant. Thus, after two weeks the elimination of host T cells, using depleting anti-human CD2, did not prevent the acceptance of second donor skin grafts.[51] These "converted" cells could then prevent a new cohort of naive T cells from rejecting the graft thus demonstrating suppression or "infectious tolerance" according to the term coined by Gershon in 1971.[53] It is important to emphasize here that in rodents, especially mice, skin allografting represents the most arduous transplantation model and one in which robust tolerance is difficult to achieve. Less aggressive immunosuppressive treatments seem to be needed, irrespective of the H-2 disparity, for models such as vascularized heart allografts or endocrine non-vascularized tissue allografts i.e., thyroid implants or islet of Langerhans. In such experimental models various depleting or non depleting antibodies to CD4, used and applied alone for very short treatment courses at the time of transplant, promoted prolonged graft survival.[54-57]

Interestingly enough, mice recipients of cardiac allografts treated with short perioperative course of antibodies to CD4 will develop at about 2 months post-transplant a state of antigen-specific tolerance in that they will accept indefinitely skin grafts matched to the heart donor, but will reject acutely third party skin grafts.[58] Nevertheless, during the initial phase, i.e., the 2-month period needed to establish tolerance, the effect of anti-CD4 treatment is that of non-specific immunosuppression.[59]

With the aim of devising strategies that would promote a fully operational specific tolerance state at the time of transplantation, pretransplantion conditioning regimens, combining anti-CD4 with donor histocompatibility antigens in the form of whole blood transfusion, have been tested.[58] This has resulted in 70% long term graft survival and needs a minimum interval of 4 weeks between conditioning and transplantation. Moreover, tolerance can be maintained by rechallenge at regular intervals with donor whole blood alone allowing an indefinite delay in transplantation. The potential clinical applicability of this type of protocol is evident and preliminary trials are in progress combining variably matched blood transfusion and anti-human CD4 as a conditioning regimen pretransplantation (PJ Morris, personal communication).

Despite the fact that most studies concerning tolerance induction to organ allografts have focused on antibodies to CD4, other specificities also deserve interest, for instance, antibodies to CD3, the combination of antibodies to LFA-1 and ICAM-1 and antibodies to CD25 (especially in rat transplant models).

Isobe et al have obtained very interesting results showing that combined administration of LFA-1 and ICAM-1 to mice not only resulted in permanent engraftment of fully mismatched vascularised heart allografts but also specific tolerance to donor type skin allografts.[8] However, it is important to stress that targeting other pairs of adhesion molecules may not have the same type of effect. The results of blocking CD2/LFA-3 interactions have been largely disappointing. Antibodies to CD2 may interfere with immune responses in mice, but no relevant effects on in vivo allogeneic responses (graft rejection) have been obtained.[60,61] Studies in monkeys have had similarly disappointing results.[62] Recently a synergistic effect between monoclonal antibodies to CD2 and CD3 has been described, but needs confirmation.[63]

Quite unexpected new data has shown that antibodies to CD3 can promote long-term specific unresponsiveness to autoantigens and alloantigens. Thus, in NOD (non-obese diabetic) mice, who develop a spontaneous T-cell-mediated autoimmune insulin-dependent diabetes mellitus, a shortcourse of low-dose anti-CD3 at the overt disease stage induces permanent remission.[16] Similarly, in the rat, anti-CD3 treatment leads to permanent engraftment of histoincompatible vascularized heart grafts and permanent tolerance (skin graft acceptance).[64]

The precise immune mechanisms mediating permanent engraftment and tolerance in antibody-treated adult recipients is poorly understood. One important difference with the neonatal tolerance model is that in adult recipients tolerance coexists with the presence of detectable alloreactive cells, i.e. there is no evidence for massive clonal deletion. In several of the models already described, alloreactive cells are present in the periphery of tolerant animals or even within or in the vicinity of the tolerated allograft.[57]

Although in vivo such infiltrating cells are not harmful to the allograft, in vitro they may exhibit conventional cytotoxic capacities, a condition defined as "split-tolerance." Thus, at variance with the developing immune system in which clonal deletion plays a central role, in the adult host other mechanisms predominate, the molecular bases of which are still ill-defined. These may include anergy, suppression, vetoing, cytokine-mediated immune deviation or network regulation.[4]

Peripheral immune cells which are specifically unresponsive to antigen stimulation but sensitive to non-specific signaling are termed anergic. Several different pathways which could result in T-cell anergy have been described. According to in vitro data first reported by R. Schwartz's group, anergy may result from the exclusive engagement of the T-cell receptor in the absence of costimulatory signals.[65] In the case of naive T cells, evidence suggests that CD28/CTLA4 receptors on lymphocytes and the B7 antigens on antigen presenting cells represents a fundamental costimulatory pathway.[10, 66-70] In the case of primed T cells, signals provided through the interaction of CD4 or CD8 with major histocompatibility molecules, the ligation of adhesion molecules (LFA-1/ICAM-1) and/or the effect of cytokines all may contribute to provide costimulatory signals.

In vivo, the use of transgenic animals has revealed that T-cell unresponsiveness may be related to marked down-regulation of the TCR and its coreceptors (i.e. CD8) on encounter with an antigen.[71,72] Double trangenic mice (H-2^{dxk}), with T cells expressing a Kb-specific TCR and hepatocytes expressing the allogeneic major histocompatibility alloantigen Kb (under the control of a liver-specific inducible promoter), were tolerant to Kb in that they did not reject Kb skin grafts.[71,72] In these animals, the degree of down-regulation of the TCR on in vivo anergic CD8$^+$ reactive cells was dependent on the amount of antigen expressed. These authors have proposed that tolerance induction is a "multi-step" process which, depending on the nature of the antigen and its site of expression, may result in a "subtle" to a deeper state of unresponsiveness in reactive cells, the ultimate step being deletion (which may also operate in the periphery).[71,72] Consistent with this hypothesis is recent data showing that cells displaying split-tolerance, i.e. in vivo but not in vitro unresponsiveness, may also become unresponsive in vitro following further adequate encounter with the antigen.[72]

Above we have detailed the principal models in which clear evidence for the existence of classical T-cell-mediated suppression has been found. Among the components of the immune system that may be involved in "suppressive" immunoregulation there is a great deal of interest in defining the exact role of cytokines. Cytokines are essential mediators of immunity and inflammation, two mechanisms that operate to variable extents during each of the three essential phases of the alloimmune response, i.e., antigen recognition, proliferation and differentiation of committed cells and, finally, target destruction. Cytokine-producing T cells are heterogeneous, and both in rodents and humans two major subsets of CD4⁺ cells (TH1 and TH2) with distinct cytokine-producing patterns can be distinguished. TH1 cells essentially secrete IL-2 and IFNγ and are implicated in cellular-mediated immunity, whereas TH2 cells are IL-4, IL-5, IL-6 and IL-10 producers and are essential for humoral-mediated responses.[73] Some of these cytokines play a key role in defining the TH1/TH2 balance, since they mediate the reciprocal inhibition of the two subsets.[73] This is the case with IFNγ, which is produced by TH1 cells and inhibits TH2 cell proliferation; and also with IL-10, which is produced by TH2 cells and inhibits TH1 cell function. IL-12 produced by monocyte/macrophages has been recently shown to be important in driving the response towards TH1. Moreover, the presence of IL-4 at the time of antigen triggering may be essential in shifting the balance towards TH2. When applied to transplantation immunopathology, the raw concept that has emerged is that transplant rejection results from a preferential immune deviation towards a TH1 phenotype (i.e. IL-2 and IFNγ-producing cells predominating) and consequently may be controlled by shifting the balance towards TH2. As a consequence, much effort has been devoted to studying the role of "inhibitory" TH2 type cytokines, i.e., IL-4, IL-10 in the various tolerance models described, in particular those involving classical suppression.[51] At present, no definite conclusion can be drawn and available data suggests that this working hypothesis may be too simplistic to encompass all the subtle in vivo interactions involved in the control of alloimmunity.

An alternative model implicating anergic cells in transferable tolerance has been proposed by Lechler.[74] Human T-cell clones were rendered anergic by incubation with anti-CD3 or a specific peptide in the absence of antigen-presenting cells (APCs). These anergic cells inhibited the in vitro function of reactive cells, showing the same or a different specificity, provided the same APC was presenting the peptides specific for both partners. Competition for the APC surface and locally produced IL-2 have been proposed as the mechanisms for this effect while excluding a role for "inhibitory" cytokines (i.e. IL-4, IL-10) secreted by the anergic cells.[74]

In conclusion, it is important to stress that although further work needs to be done to clarify the molecular mechanisms, T-cell-mediated suppression represents a field that cannot be ignored by groups attempting to achieve successful clinical immuno-manipulation.

SECOND GENERATION MONOCLONAL ANTIBODIES

As a result of the remarkable progress achieved in molecular engineering of rodent monoclonal antibodies, humanized antibodies are now available. These second generation monoclonal antibodies, both chimeric and fully reshaped complementarity determining region (CDR)-grafted, show very limited immunogenicity as compared to the parental molecules.[75-78] In chimeric antibodies the constant Fc portion of the parental antibody is replaced by a human Fc. In CDR-grafted antibodies only the xenogeneic hypervariable regions determining the antigen specificity are kept.

The "humanization" of monoclonal antibodies offers several advantages aside from reduced immunogenicity. Not surprisingly, the pharmacokinetics of humanized monoclonal antibodies are significantly prolonged compared to those of the parental rodent molecules.[77-80] Dramatically altering the biological/therapeutical potency of a monoclonal antibody can have both favorable and hazardous consequences (i.e. lower doses needed to achieve the same therapeutic effect versus, in the case of immunosuppressive monoclonal antibodies, an increased risk of overimmunosuppression). In addition, humanization also affects the immunological properties of the antibody molecule independently from its fine specificity (shared by idiotypic determinants). The selection "à la carte" of different Fc constant portions that will or will not interact with specific Fc receptors at the surface of immune or reticuloendothelial cells will, for example, determine the biodistribution of the monoclonal antibody (including trans-placental transfer), its metabolism and opsonizing/depleting capacities as well as its capacity to mediate cross-linking of targeted T-cell receptors.[81,82] For some monoclonal antibodies, effective cross-linking represents a crucial step mediating antigenic modulation of the cell target receptors and the transduction of activating/mitogenic signals.[83-86] One of the best examples illustrating this point is that of monoclonal antibodies to CD3. Contrasting with their potent immunosuppressive activity, antibodies to CD3 are unique in their capacity to induce a polyclonal monocyte-dependent T-cell activation leading to in vitro mitogenicity and in vivo massive, although transient, cytokine release (including TNF, IFNγ, IL-2, IL-3, IL-4, IL-6, IL-10 and GM CSF).[84,85,87-89] The cytokine-related acute "flu-like" syndrome associated with anti-CD3 monoclonal antibody administration is a major clinical problem (also discussed in the contribution of Abramowicz et al).[90,91] Finding a means of attenuating it is of utmost importance, since it hampers a more widespread clinical use of this highly potent immunosuppressant.[3,92,93] This reaction is monocyte dependent, as illustrated, firstly by the variability of the in vitro and in vivo response, depending on the murine antibody isotype (IgG2a >> IgG1 >> IgG2b >>> IgA) corresponding to the variable affinity of human monocyte Fc receptors for murine IgG isotypes[84,85,94,95] and secondly, by the lack of response with F(ab')2 fragments.[16,85,96]

Not surprisingly, there is great interest in the development of "non-activating" antibodies to CD3, expressing constant Fc portions that do not interact with monocyte receptors; as is the case for mouse IgA and some humanized antibodies.[82,94,95,97]

A major mode of action of anti-CD3 monoclonal antibodies is antigenic modulation, i.e., reversible disappearance of a given cell receptor following binding of a specific ligand, resulting in microaggregation of the complex, capping and subsequent internalization or shedding.[83,98,99] In mice given doses of anti-CD3 comparable to those used in the clinic, only 30-40% of CD3+ cells are actually depleted via non complement-dependent routes (phagocytosis secondary to opsonisation, apoptosis and bystander cell killing).[16,100-103] The remaining cells undergo specific antigenic modulation of their CD3/TCR receptor (i.e. CD3-TCR-CD4+ or CD3-TCR-CD8+). These appear in small but nevertheless significant numbers in both the circulation and amongst cells infiltrating the allograft when OKT3 is used to treat acute rejection.[98,104-106] These antigenically-modulated cells are unresponsive to mitogens and alloantigens which explains the absence of detectable clinical allograft rejection in patients undergoing effective OKT3 treatment.[3,98,99] F(ab')2 fragments of anti-CD3 have shown therapeutic capacities comparable to the whole antibody when used in rodent transplant and autoimmune models.[16,96] In both settings F(ab´)2 fragments promoted a dose-dependent antigenic modulation of the CD3/TCR that was however less pronounced and long-lasting than that observed with the whole antibody molecule.[16,96] This is in keeping with published, although not entirely confirmed, in vitro data showing that monocytes are required to achieve effective anti-CD3-mediated antigenic modulation.

A fundamental question, still open to debate, is whether antigenic modulation of CD3/TCR correlates and/or is indispensable for the in vivo therapeutic capacity of antibodies to CD3. Two monoclonal antibodies to monomorphic TCR determinants BMA-031, a mouse IgG2b, and T10B9.1A-31 (mouse IgM), have been tested in controlled clinical trials. Although they appear to have similar biological effects to OKT3, i.e., some T-cell depletion linked to opsonization and a large proportion of T cells with antigenically modulated CD3/TCRs,[107-113] they seem to be far less immunosuppressive as evidenced not only by the transplants course but also by the rapid rise in high titer specific anti-idiotypic neutralizing antibodies.[109-113] This data suggests that antigenic modulation per se does not necessarily correlate with the in vivo therapeutic capacity of a monoclonal antibody. What probably matters is the transduction of adequate signaling upon antibody binding to its receptor as well as the fate of internalized receptor-antibody complexes.

Interestingly enough, the cytolytic capacity of some monoclonal antibodies can be improved by means other than manipulation of the Fc domains. Recently a monovalent antibody to CD3 has been derived by somatic cell fusion of the anti-CD3-producing hybridoma with another Ig-producing cell line. In the presence of human complement, this antibody is far more lytic than the parent bivalent rat antibody.[114] This improved lytic potential is not explicable in terms of a difference in complement activation (i.e. C1q binding or cell-associated C3). In a preliminary clinical trial, the use of this monovalent anti-CD3 was shown to be safe. At variance to OKT3, no first-dose side effects were observed and in terms of reversal of established acute renal allograft rejection the clinical data is encouraging (Abbs I, personal communication).

ADDITIONAL REMARKS ON SENSITIZATION

When the first clinical trials were started, the high immunogenicity of monoclonal antibodies was quite unexpected. In fact, compared to polyclonal reagents (ATG or ALG preparations), monoclonal antibodies represented homogeneous sets of highly purified, mostly deaggregated, immunoglobulins injected i.v. which is considered as a low immunogenic route. The immune response elicited by monoclonal antibodies, independently from their fine specificity, is far from massive due to its exquisite restriction in clonality and fine specificity, with only anti-isotypic and anti-idiotypic antibodies being produced.[44,104,115] This probably explains why the clinical consequences of the sensitization to monoclonal antibodies differs significantly from that observed with conventional polyclonal preparations. Immune complex disease in general and serum sickness in particular have never been reported among the thousands of patients treated with OKT3. This does not mean it cannot occur, since specific immune complexes do form and can be identified in the serum of immunized patients undergoing monoclonal antibody treatment (L. Chatenoud, unpublished data). However, with conventional therapeutic protocols, immune complexes seem to be rapidly cleared without eliciting harmful reactions secondary to tissue deposition. Neutralization of the monoclonal antibody's therapeutic activity is in fact the main consequence of sensitization irrespective of the antibody fine specificity. Although this humoral response can be significantly reduced in adult patients by adequate cover with conventional immunosuppressants it remains a clinically relevant problem when retreatment with the same antibody is needed or in clinical settings other than transplantation, i.e., autoimmune diseases where, for obvious reasons, there is reluctance to introduce more than one heavy immunosuppressant at a time. Pediatric patients must be considered separately; sensitization to OKT3 is more intense in transplanted children and in contrast to adults they do not respond favorably to combined immunosuppressants.[116]

The neutralizing potential of the humoral response to xenogeneic monoclonals is entirely linked to the presence of IgG anti-idiotypic antibodies that actively compete for the binding to the target.[44,104,115,117,118] It is interesting to recall here that, according to data first reported by Benjamin et al, the anti-idiotypic component of the response is quantitatively more important and more resistant to tolerance-induction protocols in the case of "cell binding" as compared to "non-cell binding" antibodies.[44] The fact that humanized antibodies have reduced immunogenicity, despite the continued expression of idiotypic xenogeneic determinants, strongly suggests that helper epitopes driving the "carrier" effect are concentrated within the murine Fc constant regions. This is consistent with the finding that there are no major differences between the sensitizing potential of chimeric and fully reshaped humanized antibodies.[77-80] However, of particular relevance for future use of monoclonal antibodies is that repeated treatment with the same humanized monoclonal antibody can result in sensitization to idiotypic and allotypic determinants.[78-80,119]

The last point deserving attention is that IgE-mediated hypersensitivity responses have turned out to be very infrequent in patients sensitized to monoclonal antibodies (see chapter by Abramowicz et al).

ADDITIONAL APPLICATIONS OF THERAPEUTIC MONOCLONAL ANTIBODIES

As illustrated by other contributors to this book, monoclonal antibodies have until now been used essentially as immunosuppressive agents in organ transplantation. However, there are other fields in which they may become applicable in the foreseeable future. For example, protection against infectious agents still represents a major clinical challenge. A number of experimental models indicate potential protective uses for monoclonal antibodies to bacteria or viruses. The old concept of serotherapy could thus be revisited if the "active" monoclonal or oligoclonal immunoglobulin components of the "protective" sera were characterized. This approach could prove particularly useful in cytomegalovirus and cocsackie virus infections. Data recently reported on patients presenting with the acquired immunodeficiency syndrome (AIDS), who were passively transfused with high titer anti-HIV antibody containing sera from asymptomatic seropositive patients, further supports the importance of this type of approach, especially in situations where no specific vaccine exists.[120] Another strategy, applicable in combating viral infections, is to target the specific receptor allowing cell penetration. Thus, in heavily immunosuppressed patients, the progression of massive Epstein-Barr virus (EBV)-induced lymphoproliferation has been successfully arrested using monoclonal antibodies to CD21 and CD24.[121,122]

The targeting of costimulatory pathways represents another interesting field. As already mentioned, T cells require two signals for activation: signal 1 is provided by stimulation through the TCR, and signal 2 (the "costimulatory" signal) is provided by ligation of one or more T-cell surface receptors. Engagement of TCR alone, i.e. delivery of signal 1 without signal 2, promotes T-cell-specific unresponsiveness (anergy).[65] The first costimulatory pathway to be characterized was that transduced through the CD28 molecule, whose specific ligand B7/BB1 is present at the surface of antigen-presenting cells.[10,66-70] CTLA-4 is the product of a gene closely related to CD28, that also acts as a B7 ligand. A recently described soluble recombinant fusion protein, CTLA-4Ig, effectively competed for CD28 engagement and blocked T-cell-dependent responses in vitro. In vivo, CTLA4Ig is immunosuppressive: it can block T-cell-dependent antibody production and prevent pancreatic islet xenograft and allogeneic cardiac allograft rejection.[10,69,70] Whether CTLA4Ig, when used alone, is able to promote long-term graft acceptance is still open to debate.

Finally, in some clinical situations, cytokine neutralization may be useful. To neutralize the biological effect of cytokines, one must inhibit their binding to specific receptors. In theory, this can be achieved in various ways, including treatment with anti-cytokine antibodies, soluble cytokine receptors, antagonists of cytokine receptors (as in the case of IL-1) and genetically engineered immunoadhesins, including two soluble receptor fragments linked to an immunoglobulin constant frame.[123-128] Given the variable pharmacodynamic behavior of cytokine-binding molecules, in that they can behave both as agonists and antagonists, achieving cytokine neutralization is more difficult than it would first appear. This is illustrated by the effect of anti-IL-6, anti-IL-3, anti-IL-4 and anti-IL-7 monoclonal antibodies who, far from enhancing clearance of the target cytokine, act as in vivo carrier proteins and thereby prolong the half-life and enhance the biological effects of their ligand.[129-132]

There are two distinct pathological settings in which therapeutic strategies aimed at cytokine neutralization may be beneficial. The first involves diseases due to over-production of a given cytokine; e.g., acute inflammation, sepsis and cytokine-dependent tumor growth (e.g., multiple myeloma).[132,133] The second setting comprises conditions such as allograft rejection, that involve immunologically-mediated target tissue damage which may be highly sensitive, as already discussed, to the regulatory effect of some key TH1- or TH2-derived cytokines (i.e. IFNγ, IL-4, IL-10, IL-12). A TH1/TH2 shift has been obtained in vivo by means such as anti-cytokine antibodies (anti-IFNγ, anti-IL-4),[134] anti-T-cell antibodies (especially anti-CD4 at low doses) and delivery of the cytokines themselves, e.g., IL-4 or IL-10. Time will tell whether such attractive immunomodulatory means may be effectively applied in clinical transplantation.

Proinflammatory cytokines such as tumor necrosis factor (TNF), interleukin-1β (IL-1β) and IL-6 are also induced during rejection and participate in target damage through their effect on vessels (vasodilatation, increased vascular permeability and endothelial activation), coagulation (increased pro-coagulant capacity, thrombosis and hemorrhage) and permissive effects on cell infiltration (chemotactic activity). Some authors claim that antibodies to TNF can prolong allograft survival.[135,136] Potentially interesting as these results are, they still need confirmation.

CONCLUSION

With the development of humanized monoclonal antibodies, their potential therapeutic uses are set to expand. Already they have spread from the field of transplantation to the fields of autoimmunity, infectious diseases and cancer. Data on preliminary clinical trials using these antibodies to treat wide-ranging autoimmune diseases are now beginning to emerge; non-depleting CD4 monoclonals have been used to treat psoriasis, unresponsive to other conventional treatments, with very encouraging results,[137,138] antibodies to tumor necrosis factor (TNF) appear to have short-lived but reproducible effects in ameliorating symptoms in severe rheumatoid arthritis[79,80] and, the results of using anti-CD52 (CAMPATH-1G) to treat relentlessly progressive, life-threatening Wegener's granulomatosis are impressive.[119] Monoclonal antibodies against specific tumor antigens are being studied with the aim of directing the cytolytic response against unmodified malignant cells, avoiding both the destruction of healthy tissue and the severe generalized immunosuppression that accompanies current treatments.[139] It is easy to imagine the role these antibodies could play in destroying microscopic metastasis after the main tumor has been surgically debulked.[139]

The future for monoclonal antibodies is exciting. Enormous progress has been made in the last 15 years and it is likely that before a similar time period has elapsed they will have become standard tools, no longer shrouded in mystery, in both transplantation and other clinical arenas. Perhaps the time will come when transplantation covered by a combination of monoclonal antibodies, constituting an ideal "oligoclonal" cocktail, will result in specific tolerance to alloantigens, dispensing with the need for long term immunosuppression with all its inherent dangers.

REFERENCES

1. Cosimi AB, Colvin RB, Burton RC et al. Use of monoclonal antibodies to T-cell subsets for immunologic monitoring and treatment in recipients of renal allografts. N Engl J Med 1981; 305:308-314.
2. Cosimi AB, Burton RC, Colvin RB et al. Treatment of acute renal allograft rejection with OKT3 monoclonal antibody. Transplantation 1981; 32:535-539.
3. Ortho Multicenter Transplant Study Group. A randomized clinical trial of OKT3 monoclonal antibody for acute rejection of cadaveric renal transplants. N Engl J Med 1985; 313:337-342.
4. Schwartz RH. Immunological tolerance. In: Fundamental Immunology, Paul WE (Ed.) 1993; 677-731.
5. Benjamin RJ, Waldmann H. Induction of tolerance by monoclonal antibody therapy. Nature 1986; 320:449-451.
6. Gutstein NL, Seaman WE, Scott JH et al. Induction of immune tolerance by administration of monoclonal antibody to L3T4. J Immunol 1986; 137:1127-1132.
7. Cobbold SP, Qin S, Leong LY et al. Reprogramming the immune system for peripheral tolerance with CD4 and CD8 monoclonal antibodies. Immunol Rev 1992; 129:165-201.
8. Isobe M, Yagita H, Okumura K et al. Specific acceptance of cardiac allograft after treatment with antibodies to ICAM-1 and LFA-1. Science 1992; 255:1125-1127.
9. Springer TA, Dustin ML, Kishimoto TK et al. The lymphocyte function-associated LFA-1, CD2, and LFA-3 molecules: cell adhesion receptors of the immune system. Annu Rev Immunol 1987; 5:223-252.
10. Lin H, Bolling SF, Linsley PS et al. Long-term acceptance of major histocompatibility complex mismatched cardiac allografts induced by CTLA4Ig plus donor-specific transfusion. J Exp Med 1993; 178:1801-1806.

11. Brostoff SW, Mason DW. Experimental allergic encephalomyelitis: successful treatment in vivo with a monoclonal antibody that recognizes T helper cells. J Immunol 1984; 133:1938-1942.
12. Christadoss P, Dauphinee MJ. Immunotherapy for myasthenia gravis: a murine model. J Immunol 1986; 136:2437-2440.
13. Wofsy D, Seaman WE. Reversal of advanced murine lupus in NZB/NZW F1 mice by treatment with monoclonal antibody to L3T4. J Immunol 1987; 138:3247-3253.
14. Waldor MK, Sriram S, Hardy R et al. Reversal of experimental allergic encephalomyelitis with monoclonal antibody to a T-cell subset marker. Science 1985; 227:415-417.
15. Shizuru JA, Taylor-Edwards C, Banks BA et al. Immunotherapy of the nonobese diabetic mouse: treatment with an antibody to T-helper lymphocytes. Science 1988; 240:659-662.
16. Chatenoud L, Thervet E, Primo J et al. Anti-CD3 antibody induces long-term remission of overt autoimmunity in nonobese diabetic mice. Proc Natl Acad Sci USA 1994; 91:123-127.
17. Schwartz RS. Autoimmunity and autoimmune diseases. In: Fundamental Immunology, Paul WE (Ed.) 1993; 1033-1097
18. Owen RD. Immunogenetic consequences of vascular anastomoses between bovine twins. Science 1945; 102:400-401.
19. Billingham RE, Brent L, Medawar PB. Actively acquired tolerance to foreign cells. Nature 1953; 172:603-606.
20. Sykes M, Sachs DH. Bone marrow transplantation as a means of inducing tolerance. Semin Immunol 1990; 2:401-417.
21. Roser BJ. Cellular mechanisms in neonatal and adult tolerance. Immunol Rev 1989; 107:179-202.
22. Heeg K, Wagner H. Analysis of immunological tolerance to major histocompatibility complex antigens. I. High frequencies of tolerogen-specific cytotoxic T lymphocyte precursors in mice neonatally tolerized to class I major histocompatibility complex antigens. Eur J Immunol 1985; 15:25-30.
23. Stockinger B. Cytotoxic T-cell precursors revealed in neonatally tolerant mice. Proc Natl Acad Sci USA 1984; 81:220-223.
24. Streilein JW, Gruchalla RS. Analysis of neonatally induced tolerance of H-2 alloantigens. I. Adoptive transfer indicates that tolerance of class I and class II antigens is maintained by distinct mechanisms. Immunogenetics 1981; 12:161-173.
25. Nossal GJ, Pike BL. Functional clonal deletion in immunological tolerance to major histocompatibility complex antigens. Proc Natl Acad Sci USA 1981; 78:3844-3847.
26. McCarthy SA, Bach FH. The cellular mechanism of maintenance of neonatally induced tolerance to H-2 class I antigens. J Immunol 1983; 131:1676-1682.
27. Speiser DE, Schneider R, Hengartner H et al. Clonal deletion of self-reactive T cells in irradiation bone marrow chimeras and neo-

natally tolerant mice. Evidence for intercellular transfer of Mlsa. J Exp Med 1989; 170:595-600.

28. Sykes M, Sheard M, Sachs DH. Effects of T cell depletion in radiation bone marrow chimeras. I. Evidence for a donor cell population which increases allogeneic chimerism but which lacks the potential to produce GVHD. J Immunol 1988; 141:2282-2288.

29. Zinkernagel RM, Althage A, Callahan G et al. On the immunocompetence of H-2 incompatible irradiation bone marrow chimeras. J Immunol 1980; 124:2356-2365.

30. Lapidot T, Terenzi A, Singer TS et al. Enhancement by dimethyl myleran of donor type chimerism in murine recipients of bone marrow allografts. Blood 1989; 73:2025-2032.

31. Leong Ly, Qin S, Cobbold SP et al. Classical transplantation tolerance in the adult: the interaction between myeloablation and immunosuppression. Eur J Immunol 1992; 22:2825-2830.

32. Deeg HJ, Storb R, Thomas ED. Bone marrow transplantation: a review of delayed complications. Br J Haematol 1984; 57:185-208.

33. Monaco AP, Wood ML, Russell PS. Studies on heterologous antilymphocyte serum in mice. III. Immunological tolerance and chimerism produced across the H2-locus with adult thymectomy and antilymphocyte serum. Ann NY Acad Sci 1966; 129:190.

34. Wood ML, Monaco AP, Gozzo JJ et al. Use of homozygous allogeneic bone marrow for induction of tolerance with antilymphocyte serum: dose and timing. Transplant Proc 1971; 3:676-679.

35. Maki T, Gottschalk R, Wood ML et al. Specific unresponsiveness to skin allografts in anti-lymphocyte serum-treated, marrow-injected mice: participation of donor marrow-derived suppressor T cells. J Immunol 1981; 127:1433-1438.

36. Bobbio SA, Wood ML, Monaco AP. Significant augmentation of specific unresponsiveness by rapamycin in ALS-treated, bone marrow injected mice. Transplant Sci 1993; 3:51-55.

37. Thomas JM, Carver FM, Foil MB et al. Renal allograft tolerance induced with ATG and donor bone marrow in outbred rhesus monkeys. Transplantation 1983; 36:104-106.

38. Thomas J, Carver M, Cunningham P et al. Promotion of incompatible allograft acceptance in rhesus monkeys given posttransplant antithymocyte globulin and donor bone marrow. I. In vivo parameters and immunohistologic evidence suggesting microchimerism. Transplantation 1987; 43:332-338.

39. Thomas JM, Carver FM, Cunningham PR et al. Kidney allograft tolerance in primates without chronic immunosuppression—the role of veto cells. Transplantation 1991; 51:198-207.

40. Thomas J, Alqaisi M, Cunningham P et al. The development of a posttransplant TLI treatment strategy that promotes organ allograft acceptance without chronic immunosuppression. Transplantation 1992; 53:247-258.

41. Miller RG. The veto phenomenom and T cell regulation. Immunol Today 1986; 7:112-114.
42. Wofsy D, Mayes DC, Woodcock J et al. Inhibition of humoral immunity in vivo by monoclonal antibody to L3T4: studies with soluble antigens in intact mice. J Immunol 1985; 135:1698-1701.
42. Wolfsy D, Mayes DC, Woodcock J, Seaman EW. Inhibition of humoral immunity in vivo by monoclonal antibody to L3T4: studies with soluble antigens in intact mice. J Immunol 1985; 135:1698-1701.
43. Goronzy J, Weyand CM, Fathman CG. Long-term humoral unresponsiveness in vivo, induced by treatment with monoclonal antibody against L3T4. J Exp Med 1986; 164:911-925.
44. Benjamin RJ, Cobbold SP, Clark MR et al. Tolerance to rat monoclonal antibodies. Implications for serotherapy. J Exp Med 1986; 163:1539-1552.
45. Benjamin RJ, Qin SX, Wise MP et al. Mechanisms of monoclonal antibody-facilitated tolerance induction: a possible role for the CD4 (L3T4) and CD11a (LFA-1) molecules in self-non-self discrimination. Eur J Immunol 1988; 18:1079-1088.
46. Qin S, Cobbold S, Tighe H et al. CD4 monoclonal antibody pairs for immunosuppression and tolerance induction. Eur J Immunol 1987; 17:1159-1165.
47. Gutstein NL, Wofsy D. Administration of F(ab')2 fragments of monoclonal antibody to L3T4 inhibits humoral immunity in mice without depleting L3T4+ cells. J Immunol 1986; 137:3414-3419.
48. Qin SX, Wise M, Cobbold SP et al. Induction of tolerance in peripheral T cells with monoclonal antibodies. Eur J Immunol 1990; 20:2737-2745.
49. Hirsch R, Chatenoud L, Gress RE et al. Suppression of the humoral response to anti-CD3 monoclonal antibody. Transplantation 1989; 47:853-857.
50. Qin SX, Cobbold S, Benjamin R et al. Induction of classical transplantation tolerance in the adult. J Exp Med 1989; 169:779-794.
51. Qin S, Cobbold SP, Pope H et al. "Infectious" transplantation tolerance. Science 1993; 259:974-977.
52. Cobbold SP, Qin SX, Waldmann H. Reprogramming the immune system for tolerance with monoclonal antibodies. Semin Immunol 1990; 2:377-387.
53. Gershon RK, Kondo K. Infectious immunological tolerance. Immunology 1971; 21:903-914.
54. Shizuru JA, Gregory AK, Chao CT et al. Islet allograft survival after a single course of treatment of recipient with antibody to L3T4. Science 1987; 237:278-280.
55. Shizuru JA, Seydel KB, Flavin TF et al. Induction of donor-specific unresponsiveness to cardiac allografts in rats by pretransplant anti-CD4 monoclonal antibody therapy. Transplantation 1990;

50:366-373.

56. Madsen JC, Peugh WN, Wood KJ et al. The effect of anti-L3T4 monoclonal antibody treatment on first-set rejection of murine cardiac allografts. Transplantation 1987; 44:849-852.

57. Siegling A, Lehmann M, Riedel H et al. A nondepleting anti-rat CD4 monoclonal antibody that suppresses T helper 1-like but not T helper 2-like intragraft lymphokine secretion induces long-term survival of renal allografts. Transplantation 1994; 57:464-467.

58. Pearson TC, Madsen JC, Larsen CP et al. Induction of transplantation tolerance in adults using donor antigen and anti-CD4 monoclonal antibody. Transplantation 1992; 54:475-483.

59. Wood KJ. Transplantation tolerance with monoclonal antibodies. Semin Immunol 1990; 2:389-399.

60. Guckel B, Berek C, Lutz M et al. Anti-CD2 antibodies induce T cell unresponsiveness in vivo. J Exp Med 1991; 174:957-967.

61. Bromberg JS, Chavin KD, Altevogt P et al. Anti-CD2 monoclonal antibodies alter cell-mediated immunity in vivo. Transplantation 1991; 51:219-225.

62. Jonker M, Golsdstein G, Balner H. Effects of in vivo administration of monoclonal antibodies specific for human T cell subpopulations on the immune system in a rhesus monkey model. Transplantation 1983; 35:521-526.

63. Chavin KD, Qin L, Lin J et al. Combination anti-CD2 and anti-CD3 monoclonal antibodies induce tolerance while altering interleukin-2, interleukin-4, tumor necrosis factor, and transforming growth factor-beta production. Ann Surg 1993; 218:492-501.

64. Nicolls MR, Aversa GG, Pearce NW et al. Induction of long-term specific tolerance to allografts in rats by therapy with an anti-CD3-like monoclonal antibody. Transplantation 1993; 55:459-468.

65. Schwartz RH. A cell culture model for T lymphocyte clonal anergy. Science 1990; 248:1349-1356.

66. Linsley PS, Clark EA, Ledbetter JA. T-cell antigen CD28 mediates adhesion with B cells by interacting with activation antigen B7/BB-1. Proc Natl Acad Sci USA 1990; 87:5031-5035.

67. Linsley PS, Brady W, Urnes M et al. CTLA-4 is a second receptor for the B cell activation antigen B7. J Exp Med 1991; 174:561-569.

68. Van Den Eertwegh AJ, Noelle RJ, Roy M et al. In vivo CD40-gp39 interactions are essential for thymus-dependent humoral immunity. I. In vivo expression of CD40 ligand, cytokines, and antibody production delineates sites of cognate T-B cell interactions. J Exp Med 1993; 178:1555-1565.

69. Linsley PS, Wallace PM, Johnson J et al. Immunosuppression in vivo by a soluble form of the CTLA-4 T cell activation molecule. Science 1992; 257:792-795.

70. Lenschow DJ, Zeng Y, Thistlethwaite JR et al. Long-term survival

of xenogeneic pancreatic islet grafts induced by CTLA4lg. Science 1992; 257:789-792.

71. Ferber I, SChonrich G, Schenkel J et al. Levels of peripheral T cell tolerance induced by different doses of tolerogen. Science 1994; 263:674-676.

72. Schonrich G, Alferink J, Klevenz et al. Tolerance induction as a multi-step process. Eur J Immunol 1994; 24:285-293.

73. Mosmann TR, Coffman RL. TH1 and TH2 cells: different patterns of lymphokine secretion lead to different functional properties. Annu Rev Immunol 1989; 7:145-173.

74. Lombardi G, Sidhu S, Batchelor R et al. Anergic T cells as suppressor cells in vitro. Science 1994; 264:1587-1589.

75. Morrison SL, Johnson MJ, Herzenberg LA et al. Chimeric human antibody molecules: mouse antigen-binding domains with human constant region domains. Proc Natl Acad Sci USA 1984; 81:6851-6855.

76. Riechmann L, Clark M, Waldmann H et al. Reshaping human antibodies for therapy. Nature 1988; 332:323-327.

77. Lazarovits AI, Rochon J, Banks L et al. Human mouse chimeric CD7 monoclonal antibody (SDZCHH380) for the prophylaxis of kidney transplant rejection. J Immunol 1993; 150:5163-5174.

78. Isaacs JD, Watts RA, Hazleman BL et al. Humanised monoclonal antibody therapy for rheumatoid arthritis. Lancet 1992; 340:748-752.

79. Elliot MJ, Maini RN, Feldmann M et al. Randomised double-blind comparison of chimeric monoclonal antibody to tumour necrosis factor alpha (cA2) versus placebo in rheumatoid arthritis. Lancet 1994; 344:1105-1110.

80. Elliot MJ, Maini RN, Feldmann M et al. Repeated therapy with monoclonal antibody to tumour necrosis factor alpha (cA2) in patients with rheumatoid arthritis. Lancet 1994; 344:1125-1127.

81. Isaacs JD, Clark MR, Greenwood J et al. Therapy with monoclonal antibodies. An in vivo model for the assessment of therapeutic potential. J Immunol 1992; 148:3062-3071.

82. Bolt S, Routledge E, Lloyd I et al. The generation of a humanized, non-mitogenic CD3 monoclonal antibody which retains in vitro immunosuppressive properties. Eur J Immunol 1993; 23:403-411.

83. Chatenoud L, Bach JF. Antigenic modulation: a major mechanism of antibody action. Immunol Today 1984; 5:20-25.

84. Van Lier RA, Boot, de Groot ER et al. Induction of T cell proliferation with anti-CD3 switch-variant monoclonal antibodies: effects of heavy chain isotype in monocyte-dependent systems. Eur J Immunol 1987; 17:1599-1604.

85. Van Wauwe JP, de Mey Jr, Goossens JG. OKT3: a monoclonal anti-human T lymphocyte antibody with potent mitogenic properties. J Immunol 1980; 124:2708-2713.

86. Emmrich F, Kanz L, Eichmann K. Cross-linking of the T cell receptor complex with the subset-specific differentiation antigen stimulates interleukin 2 receptor expression in human CD4 and CD8 T cells. Eur J Immunol 1987; 17:529-534.
87. Chatenoud L, Ferran C, Legendre C et al. In vivo cell activation following OKT3 administration. Systemic cytokine release and modulation by corticosteroids. Transplantation 1990; 49:697-702.
88. Abramowicz D, Schandene L, Goldmann M et al. Release of tumor necrosis factor, interleukin-2, and gamma-interferon in serum after injection of OKT3 monoclonal antibody in kidney transplant recipients. Transplantation 1989; 47:606-608.
89. Ferran C, Dy M, Sheehan K et al. Cascade modulation by antitumor necrosis factor monoclonal antibody of interferon-gamma, interleukin 3 and interleukin 6 release after triggering of the CD3/T cell receptor activation pathway. Eur J Immunol 1991; 21:2349-2353.
90. Chatenoud L, Legendre C, Ferran C et al. Corticosteroid inhibition of the OKT3-induced cytokine-related syndrome—dosage and kinetics prerequisites. Transplantation 1991; 51:334-338.
91. Charpentier B, Hiesse C, Lantz O et al. Evidence that antihuman tumor necrosis factor monoclonal antibody prevents OKT3-induced acute syndrome. Transplantation 1992; 54:997-1002.
92. Cosimi AB. Clinical development of Orthoclone OKT3. Transplant Proc 1987; 19:7-16.
93. Goldstein G. Overview of the development of Orthoclone OKT3: monoclonal antibody for therapeutic use in transplantation. Transplant Proc 1987; 19:1-6.
94. Parlevliet KJ, Jonker M, Ten Berge RJ et al. Anti-CD3 murine monoclonal isotype switch variants tested for toxicity and immunologic monitoring in four chimpanzees. Transplantation 1990; 50:889-892.
95. Parlevliet KJ, Ten Berge IJ, Yong SL et al. In vivo effects of IgA and IgG2a anti-CD3 isotype switch variants. J Clin Invest 1994; 93:2519-2525.
96. Hirsch R, Bluestone Ja, De Nenno L et al. Anti-CD3 F(ab')2 fragments are immunosuppressive in vivo without evoking either the strong humoral response or morbidity associated with whole mAb. Transplantation 1990; 49:1117-1123.
97. Alegre ML, Collins AM, Pulito VL et al. Effect of a single amino acid mutation on the activating and immunosuppressive properties of a "humanized" OKT3 monoclonal antibody. J Immunol 1992; 148:3461-3468.
98. Chatenoud L, Baudihaye MF, Kreis H et al. Human in vivo antigenic modulation induced by the anti-T cell OKT3 monoclonal antibody. Eur J Immunol 1982; 12:979-982.
99. Meuer SC, Acuto O, Hercend T et al. The human T-cell receptor.

Annu Rev Immunol 1984; 2:23-50.

100. Hirsch R, Eckhaus M, Auchincloss H Jr et al. Effects of in vivo administration of anti-T3 monoclonal antibody on T cell function in mice. I. Immunosuppression of transplantation responses. J Immunol 1988; 140:3766-3772.

101. Smith CA, Williams GT, Kingston R et al. Antibodies to CD3/T-cell receptor complex induce death by apoptosis in immature T cells in thymic cultures. Nature 1989; 337:181-184.

102. Wesselborg S, Janssen O, Kabelitz D. Induction of activation-driven death (apoptosis) in activated but not resting peripheral blood T cells. J Immunol 1993; 150:4338-4345.

103. Wong JT, Colvin RB. Selective reduction and proliferation of the CD4+ and CD8+ T cell subsets with bispecific monoclonal antibodies: evidence for inter-T cell-mediated cytolysis. Clin Immunol Immunopathol 1991; 58:236-250.

104. Chatenoud L, Baudrihaye MF, Chkoff N et al. Restriction of the human in vivo immune response against the mouse monoclonal antibody OKT3. J Immunol 1986; 137:830-838.

105. Vigeral P, Chkogg N, Chatenoud L et al. Prophylactic use of OKT3 monoclonal antibody in cadaver kidney recipients. Utilization of OKT3 as the sole immunosuppressive agent. Transplantation 1986; 41:730-733.

106. Caillat-Zucman S, Blumenfeld N, Legendre C et al. The OKT3 immunosuppressive effect. In situ antigenic modulation of human graft-infiltrating T cells. Transplantation 1990; 49:156-160.

107. Schlitt HJ, Kurrle R, Wonigeit K. T cell activation by monoclonal antibodies directed to different epitopes on the human T cell receptor/CD3 complex: evidence for two different modes of activation. Eur J Immunol 1989; 19:1649-1655.

108. Land W, Hillebrand G, Illner WD et al. First clinical experience with a new TCR/CD3-monoclonal antibody (BMA 031) in kidney transplant patients. Transpl Int 1988; 1:116-117.

109. Dendorfer U, Hillebrand G, Kasper C et al. Effective prevention of interstitial rejection crises in immunological high risk patients following renal transplantation: use of high doses of the new monoclonal antibody BMA 031. Transplant Proc 1990; 22:1789-1790.

110. Knight RJ, Kurrle R, McClain J et al. Clinical evaluation of induction immunosuppression with a murine IgG2b monoclonal antibody (BMA 031) directed toward the human alpha/beta-T cell receptor. Transplantation 1994; 57:1581-1588.

111. Chatenoud L, Ferran C, Legendre C et al. Immunological follow-up of renal allograft recipients treated with the BMA 031 (anti-TCR) monoclonal antibody. Transplant Proc 1990; 22:1787-1788.

112. Chatenoud L, Legendre C, Kurrle R et al. Absence of clinical symptoms following the first injection of anti-T cell receptor monoclonal antibody (BMA 031) despite isolated TNF release. Transplantation 1993; 55:443-445.

113. Waid TH, Lucas BS, Thompson JS et al. Treatment of acute cellular rejection with T10B9.1A-31 or OKT3 in renal allograft recipients. Transplantation 1992; 53:80-86.

114. Clark M, Bindon C, Dyer M et al. The improved lytic function and in vivo efficacy of monovalent monoclonal CD3 antibodies. Eur J Immunol 1989; 19:381-388.

115. Villemain F, Jonker M, Bach JF et al. Fine specificity of antibodies produced in rhesus monkeys following in vivo treatment with anti-T cell murine monoclonal antibodies. Eur J Immunol 1986; 16:945-949.

116. Niaudet P, Jean G, Broyer M et al. Anti-OKT3 response following prophylactic treatment in paediatric kidney transplant recipients. Pediatr Nephrol 1993; 7:263-267.

117. Baudihaye MF, Chatenoud L, Kreis H et al. Unusually restricted anti-isotype human immune response to OKT3 monoclonal antibody. Eur J Immunol 1984; 14:686-691.

118. Legendre C, Kreis H, Bach JF et al. Prediction of successful allograft rejection retreatment with OKT3. Transplantation 1992; 53:87-90.

119. Lockwood CM, Thiru S, Isaacs JD et al. Long-term remission of intractable systemic vasculitis with monoclonal antibody therapy. Lancet 1993; 341:1620-1622.

120. Vittecoq D, Chevret S, Morand-Joubert L et al. Passive immunotherapy in AIDS: a double-blind randomized study based on transfusions of plasma rich in anti-human immunodeficiency virus I antibodies vs. transfusions of seronegative plasma. Proc Natl Acad Sci USA 1995; 92:1195-1199.

121. Blanche S, Le Deist F, Veber F et al. Treatment of severe Epstein-Barr virus-induced polyclonal B-lymphocyte proliferation by anti-B-cell monoclonal antibodies. Two cases after HLA-mismatched bone marrow transplantation. Ann Intern Med 1988; 108:199-203.

122. Stephan Jl, Le Deist F, Blanche S et al. Treatment of central nervous system B lymphoproliferative syndrome by local infusion of a B cell-specific monoclonal antibody. Transplantation 1992; 54:246-249.

123. Fanslow WC, Sims JE, Sassenfeld H et al. Regulation of alloreactivity in vivo by a soluble form of the interleukin-1 receptor. Science 1990; 248:739-742.

124. Jacobs CA, Lynch DH, Roux ER et al. Characterization and pharmacokinetic parameters of recombinant soluble interleukin-4 receptor. Blood 1991; 77:2396-2403.

125. Ozmen L, Gribaudo G, Fountoulakis M et al. Mouse soluble IFN gamma receptor as IFN gamma inhibitor. Distribution, antigenicity, and activity after injection in mice. J Immunol 1993; 150:2698-2705.

126. Dinarello CA, Thompson RC. Blocking IL-1: interleukin 1 receptor antagonist in vivo and in vitro. Immunol Today 1991; 12:404-410.

127. Peppel K, Crawford D, Beutler B. A tumor necrosis factor (TNF) receptor-IgG heavy chain chimeric protein as a bivalent antagonist of TNF activity. J Exp Med 1991; 174:1483-1489.

128. Lesslauer W. Tabuchi H, Gentz R et al. Recombinant soluble tumor necrosis factor receptor proteins protect mice from lipopolysaccharide-induced lethality. Eur J Immunol 1991; 21:2883-2886.

129. May LT, Neta R, Moldawer LL et al. Antibodies chaperone circulating IL-6. Paradoxical effects of anti-IL-6 "neutralizing" antibodies in vivo. J Immunol 1993; 151:3225-3236.

130. Jones AT, Ziltener HJ. Enhancement of the biologic effects of interleukin-3 in vivo by anti-interleukin-3 antibodies. Blood 1993; 82:1133-1141.

131. Finkelman FD, Madden KB, Morris SC et al. Anti-cytokine antibodies as carrier proteins. Prolongation of in vivo effects of exogenous cytokines by injection of cytokine-anti-cytokine antibody complexes. J Immunol 1993; 151:1235-1244.

132. Klein B, Wijdenes J, Zhang XG et al. Murine anti-interleukin-6 monoclonal antibody therapy for a patient with plasma cell leukemia. Blood 1991; 78:1198-1204.

133. Dinarello CA. Anti-cytokine strategies. Eur Cytokine Netw 1992; 3:7-17.

134. Bach JF. Anti-gamma interferon (IFN-gamma) monoclonal antibodies. In: Monoclonal Antibodies and Peptide Therapy in Autoimmune Diseases, BACH JF (Ed.) 1993; 319-391.

135. Imaga DK, Millis JM, Olthoff et al. The role of tumor necrosis factor in allograft rejection. II. Evidence that antibody therapy against tumor necrosis factor-alpha and lymphotoxin enhances cardiac allograft survival in rats. Transplantation 1990; 50:189-193.

136. Imaga DK, Millis JM, Seu P et al. The role of tumor necrosis factor in allograft rejection. III. Evidence that anti-TNF antibody therapy prolongs allograft survival in rats with acute rejection. Transplantation 1991; 51:57-62.

137. Nicolas JF, Chamchick N, Thivolet J et al. CD4 antibody treatment of severe psoriasis. Lancet 1991; 338:321.

138. Prinz J, Braun-Falco O, Meurer M et al. Chimaeric CD4 monoclonal antibody in treatment of generalised pustular psoriasis. Lancet 1991; 338:320-321.

139. Riethmuller G, Schneider-Gadicke E, Schlimok G et al. Randomised trial of monoclonal antibody for adjuvant therapy of resected Dukes' C colorectal carcinoma. German Cancer Aid 17-1A Study Group. Lancet 1994; 343:1177-1183.

INDEX

Page numbers in italics denote figures (f) or tables (t).

MOLECULAR BIOLOGY
INTELLIGENCE UNIT
AVAILABLE AND UPCOMING TITLES

NEUROSCIENCE INTELLIGENCE UNIT

AVAILABLE AND UPCOMING TITLES

MEDICAL INTELLIGENCE UNIT

AVAILABLE AND UPCOMING TITLES

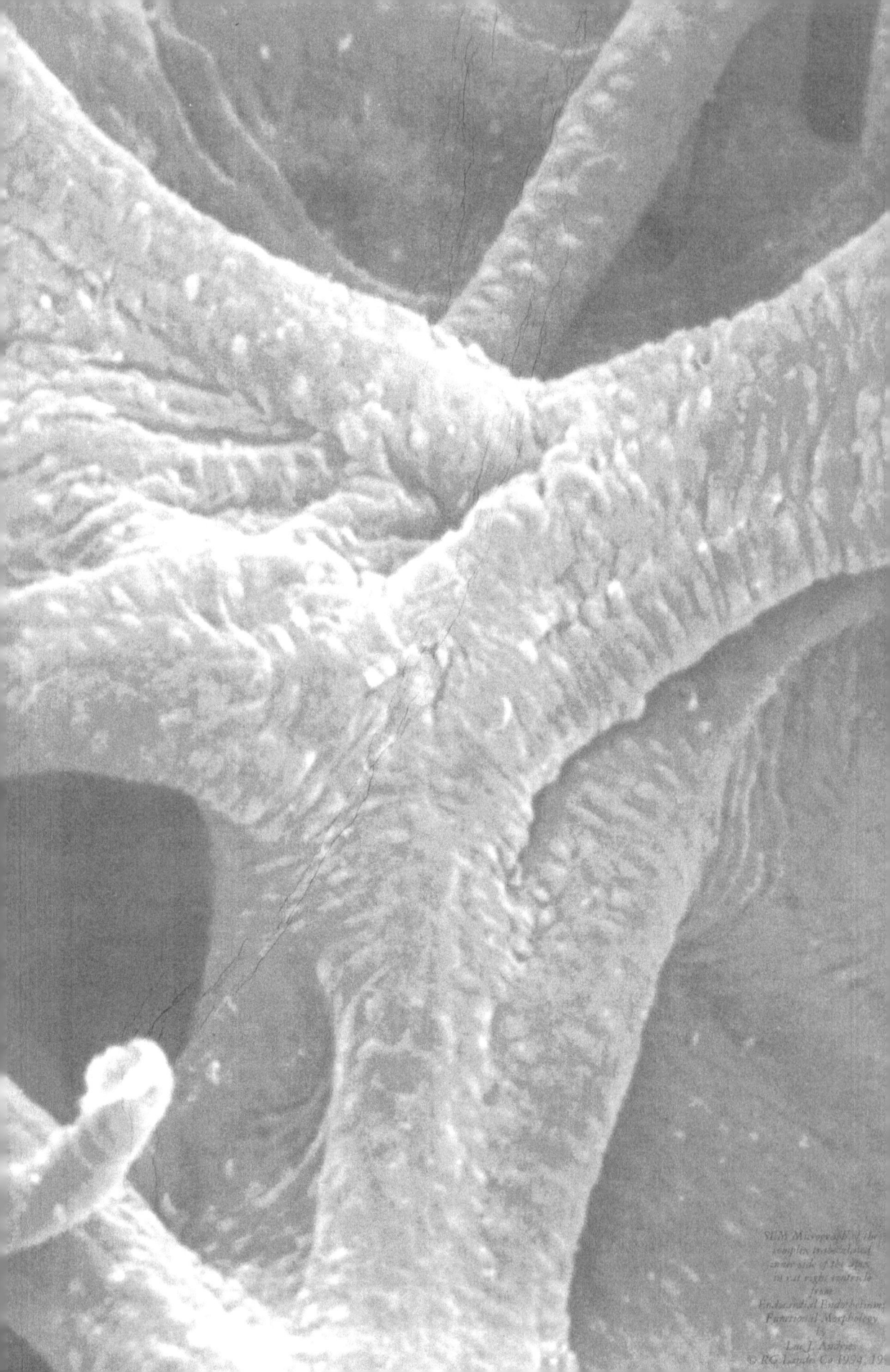